PRAISE FOR JAYNE WILLIAMS

"Williams' infectious positive attitude and her clear view of a triathlon's comic and heroic nature make *Slow Fat Triathlete* a worthy guide for everyone."

—Timothy Carlson, *Triathlon* magazine

"An inspiring, witty, and wonderfully written story that athletes of all levels can relate to. Jayne's sense of humor and confidence in herself is a breath of fresh air. There is a chuckle on every page."

—Gina Kehr, professional triathlete

"What an enjoyable book! Well-written, informative, and inspiring. Go, Jayne, go!"

—Georgena Terry, founder,
Terry Precision Bicycles for Women

"In this provocative, highly humorous, encouraging, as well as realistic and sound guide, Jayne Williams proves that anyone who really wants to can do a triathlon. Way to go, Jayne! You have crossed the finish lines of your races and your book in fine fettle."

—Steven Jonas, MD, author of
Triathloning for Ordinary Mortals and *The Essential Triathlete*

"*Slow Fat Triathlete* will get your heart-rate revved up. . . . Ideal multisport reading material for all shapes, sizes, and ages."

—Bill Katovsky, founder of *Tri-Athlete* magazine
and two-time Hawaii Ironman finisher

"*Slow Fat Triathlete* is full of practical tips and lots of funny stories about wetsuits. Williams offers her own experiences as examples to help readers get over their fear of embarrassment and failure: being the slowest runner at club training or wiping out during the swim-to-bike transition doesn't have to be a big deal. Her attitude toward unlikely but fulfilling achievements can apply beyond triathlons. Even those who pick up her book just because of its funny title may find themselves itching to try something new."

—*Harvard* magazine

"Jayne is living proof that you don't have to be young, lean, super-fit or otherwise exceptionally talented to have fun in triathlon and other endurance sports. Be prepared to laugh until coffee, or your beverage of choice, comes spurting out your nose."

—seejanerunsports.com

"Williams is the patron saint of couch potatoes, one who stead-fastly holds on to the belief that there is an athlete in all of us. You may not even have to look that hard. Throwing herself onto the bonfire of our collective vanities, Williams shares her own pilgrim-age into the world of triathlons and personal fitness. This hard-earned perspective is as insightful as it is funny. Williams is a great storyteller who insists that one need not always be the best. Instead this slow fat triathlete reminds us that there's a certain measure of satisfaction in finding the finish line on our own terms."

—*Failure* magazine

SHAPE UP

WITH THE SLOW FAT TRIATHLETE

Also by Jayne Williams

Slow Fat Triathlete:
Live Your Athletic Dreams in the Body You Have Now

SHAPE UP

WITH THE
SLOW FAT TRIATHLETE

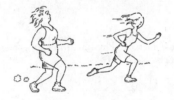

50 Ways to Kick Butt on the Field, in the Pool,
or at the Gym—No Matter What Your Size and Shape

JAYNE WILLIAMS

Da Capo
LIFE
LONG

A Member of the Perseus Books Group

Designed by Trish Wilkinson
Set in 12-point Goudy by the Perseus Books Group

Library of Congress Cataloging-in-Publication Data

Williams, Jayne, 1963–
    Shape up with the slow fat triathlete : 50 ways to kick butt on the field, in the pool, or at the gym-no matter what your size and shape / Jayne Williams. — 1st ed.
        p.   cm.
    Includes index.
    ISBN 978-1-56924-391-6 (alk. paper)
    1. Physical fitness for women. 2. Physical fitness for women—Psychological aspects.
3. Exercise. 4. Sports for women. I. Title.
GV482.W545 2009
  : 613.7'045—dc22   2008031132

First Da Capo Press edition 2009

Published by Da Capo Press
A Member of the Perseus Books Group
www.dacapopress.com

Note: The information in this book is true and complete to the best of our knowledge. This book is intended only as an informative guide for those wishing to know more about health issues. In no way is this book intended to replace, countermand, or conflict with the advice given to you by your own physician. The ultimate decision concerning care should be made between you and your doctor. We strongly recommend you follow his or her advice. Information in this book is general and is offered with no guarantees on the part of the authors or Da Capo Press. The authors and publisher disclaim all liability in connection with the use of this book.

Da Capo Press books are available at special discounts for bulk purchases in the United States by corporations, institutions, and other organizations. For more information, please contact the Special Markets Department at the Perseus Books Group, 2300 Chestnut Street, Suite 200, Philadelphia, PA 19103, or call (800) 810-4145, extension 5000, or e-mail special.markets@perseusbooks.com.

10 9 8 7 6 5 4 3 2 1

For Tim, my true North

CONTENTS

SECTION III
EIGHT WAYS TO CARE FOR YOUR BODY

SECTION IV
NINE TIPS FOR DEALING WITH
THE WORLD YOU LIVE IN

SECTION V
SEVEN ADVANCED WORKOUTS FOR YOUR MIND

SECTION VI
SEVEN PRACTICES TO INSPIRE YOUR SPIRIT

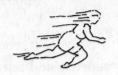

INTRODUCTION
Real Fitness
for the Rest of Us

T HIS BOOK IS for real people. Real people with jobs and
kids and love handles. Real people who dream of athleticism and joyful movement or just want to get over their horrid
flashbacks of exercise as drudgery and punishment. If you are a
regular person with ambitions of becoming more fit, but you
feel self-conscious and lumpy at the very thought of going to
the gym or donning bike shorts, this book is for you. You will
find serious, flippant, inspirational, and practical advice on how
to approach "shaping up" from a certified Slow Fat Triathlete.
Think of me not as a loud, buff, and judgmental Marine drill
instructor, but as a virtual cousin, someone who shares your imperfect genes, your challenges, and the reserves of determination and grit you may not realize you have.

First we're going to challenge, albeit gently, the fears, assumptions, hopes, and dreams that prompted you to pick up

this book. If you believe that fitness means thousands of crunches and zero cellulite; that only people like Tom Brady, Serena Williams, or Shaun Hill are really "athletes"; or that working out is anything other than pure fun, we have to shape up those thoughts in Section 1 before we can go anywhere in the physical realm.

Section 2 is about what happens when you start moving: you get hungry, sweaty, maybe uncomfortable. You get to think about how you move and whether it feels free and natural or constricted. And you get to think about whether you're bored and, if you are, how to fix that. We'll look at finding a fitness wardrobe that works (and developing a mind-set that is strong enough to be seen in Lycra, in public), the importance of your core musculature, and the joys of being outside, in water and other fun places.

Section 3 looks further at ways of caring for the wondrous system of interlocking systems that is your body and mind. We'll look at hydration, fueling, the need to protect sensitive bits of your body from chafing, and the pressing, urgent need to eat reasonable amounts of quality chocolate. We'll talk about naps, diets, doctors, and the virtues and limits of anti-inflammatory medications.

In Section 4 we think about social context and how we can reshape our thinking about it in order to become a happier athlete. We'll be looking at work, friends and family, the media, and the fitness clothing industry, as it seemingly engages in a relentless and far-ranging conspiracy to make people feel worse about their bodies than they already do.

Section 5 proposes new ways to work your brain as part of your athletic journey. Your brain is not a muscle, technically, but we're going to treat it like one, look at ways to make it get stronger as the rest of your body does the same. Do you want to embrace data but not measure your worth in terms of numbers? Paradoxical, but possible. Do you want to make the most out of your brain? Do you want to be your own superhero?

Section 6 looks at ways to inspire yourself and expand your inner resources, to get to the heights of what you can accomplish, if you want to. What do you do when life deals you a setback, or a series of them? How do you reach that mental state where worries and tension melt away as you move your body? When should you suck it up and endure, and when should you back off? How do you communicate with your body?

While I feel strongly that how you set your mind and how you believe in yourself are the most important elements of becoming an athlete, we're also going to look at bite-size, one-step-at-a-time practical tips for acquiring the habits of moving and enjoying the movement. Whether it's picking your activity of choice or paying attention to your socks, the Slow Fat Triathlete has some ideas for you.

We may think of ourselves as uncoordinated, slow, old, injured, weak, timid, fat, or some combination of the above. And all of those things may be true to some extent. I know they are for me. But if we approach an athletic endeavor, be it a triathlon, a marathon, a hiking trip, or stepping into the kickboxing ring, with insouciance, tenacity, and sheer cussedness, we can accomplish amazing things. Our bodies and our minds may be imperfect, but let's not let that get in our way. In fact, they will never be perfect—a realization I find extremely liberating.

I don't have any promises or magic bullets. What I have to offer is more realistic and more fun: a range of tips and secrets that have come in handy for me as I've made my way through a range of athletic peaks and valleys. Here are my qualifications:

I've been a couch potato with chronic injuries; I've been a fairly frequent triathlete, a slightly inexpert raft guide, a marathon finisher, an occasional rugby forward, and an annual backpacker. I enjoy shooting hoops, kicking a foot bag, swinging a bat, and diving for a football in soft sand. I read fitness literature and the odd medical paper, and I can tell my quadratus lumborum from a hole in the ground. I also enjoy talking to and learning from experts in sports and fitness, and you'll get some distillation of their wisdom along with my experiential advice.

This is a guide to fitness for all of us. I'm not one of those uber-toned personal trainers you see on the cover of other fitness books. I'm a chunky, middle-aged woman who feels strongly that everybody has the right to be an athlete, and I'm an enthusiastic cheerleader for your athleticism. I am your advocate, the voice of your athletic self urging you to bust out and move yourself about. That's what it's all about.

As an imperfect athlete, I believe you have the rights listed on the next page. So read your rights and then go out and move. And make it fun, please, because life's too short to suffer.

THE IMPERFECT ATHLETE'S BILL OF RIGHTS

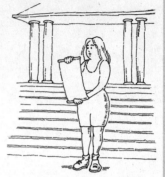

I, an imperfect athlete, hold these rights to be inalienable, and I will arm wrestle anyone who tries to deprive you of them.

You have the right to be there, no matter how much "better" than you everyone else may be.

You have the right to wear Lycra, no matter what shape your body has.

You have the right to try any sport or activity you like, at any age.

You have the right to sweat.

You have the right to develop your inner athlete, even if it sometimes inconveniences someone else's schedule.

You have the right to go as slow as you need to.

You have the right to take a nap.

You have the right to make your activity fun in whatever way you want.

You have the right to eat chocolate.

You have the right to be free of self-consciousness, everywhere and all the time.

SECTION I

NINE MODEST PROPOSALS

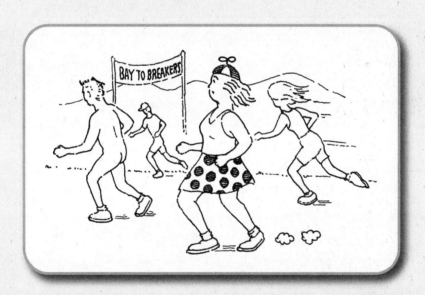

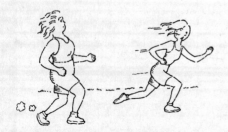

ABANDON
SELF-CONSCIOUSNESS

OKAY, PEEPS, listen up. Everything starts with this and comes back to it.

A recent study reported that 64 percent of girls and women had at some point in their lives decided not to take part in an activity because they were self-conscious about their appearance. "Argh!" I thought. I hate self-consciousness. Hate it. It's pernicious, and it comes back like dandruff. So reject it and repudiate it every gosh-darn day.

Self-consciousness is the enemy of fun, the enemy of performance, and for sure the enemy of fitness. But surely, you say, self-consciousness is actually a primary motivation for getting fit? "I need to get in shape for our vacation in tropical paradise," or "My niece is getting married in June so I have to lose fifteen pounds." You think people will be looking at you and saying, "Well heavens above, Marge, what a slob. I can't believe how some people let themselves go." So you latch onto a rigorous diet, reactivate your gym membership, and sweat your way through a routine of Stairmaster, weights, and treadmills, which you hate.

I have three issues with this scenario. Number one, you are concerned about how you look, not with getting fit. Number two, your motivation is what other people think of you. And number three, you are making exercise into drudgery on the level of emptying the cat's litter box. I'm going into all of those issues in a little bit. But this chapter is focusing on your self-consciousness (and mine; I am not immune).

Who cares what other people think? It doesn't matter one whit from the perspective of becoming a fitter, more active, happier human being. If you associate fitness with looking good in a bathing suit (and this is difficult, given prevailing cultural standards), how much fun is that going to be? Not a whole lot. And for me, fitness includes fun in a big way. Abandoning self-consciousness is the first step in the imperfect athlete's fitness program—admitting that we are imperfect and will always be so. Our bodies are not going to be golden, flawless, impossibly lean supermodel bodies. And remember that supermodels owe a lot to Photoshop.

For real people, there is no Photoshop. Even if we attain our "ideal weight," tone every muscle to its maximum potential, and achieve the cardiovascular efficiency of a Sherpa, our hips will be too wide, our calves too narrow, our feet too flat, our booties too ample. Maybe all at the same time. And yet these bodies can walk, dance, swim, climb mountains, ride a bike from Boston to New York. They can jump on a trampoline and do a downward facing dog pose. The only thing they can't do is look "perfect."

So Marge and everyone else you think will be looking at and mocking your imperfect body as you stroll along the beach or jog by on the running path also are the owners of imperfect bodies.

And they are all way too busy worrying about how they look and how other people perceive them to pay much attention to you. The few who spare a fleeting thought for you as you pass through their field of vision may have the following thoughts:

"Uh."

"Ah."

"Huh."

"Mmm . . . donut . . ."

"Oh, there goes a person. Oh, there goes another one. Oh."

"I should start jogging too."

"That chick looks like crap in a bathing suit."

What we all fear, of course, is the bathing suit comment. But there's only a 5 percent chance (based on my highly scientific calculations) that anyone is thinking about you at all, and only 16 percent of those 5 percent are thinking that you look bad. That leaves fewer than one in a hundred people with a negative thought about you, and I think you can handle that superficial, judgmental less than 1 percent. In fact, you can do more than handle it.

You can move your body and enjoy it. You can run without worrying about your breasts flopping. You can dive into the water and relish the feel of it on your skin rather than thinking about the cellulite on your thighs. You can face yourself in the mirror in the aerobics studio because you're just one more imperfect body doing your thing.

I don't pretend to have achieved a nirvana of unselfconsciousness. I am a large woman; sometimes very large, sometimes just pretty large. My bra size fluctuates between a DD and a DDD. I have a big ol' belly and a big ol' butt that jiggle and make me feel self-conscious. I have gone running after sundown so nobody could see me. I have glimpsed myself in a floor-to-ceiling mirror during a yoga class and gone "blech!" There's nothing like a downward facing dog pose to make you realize that some of your parts are hanging in directions they shouldn't.

I have decided that moving around, either outside or in the gym, is way more important than looking even halfway perfect in the eyes of anyone who happens to glance my way and think about me. Even if I get the dreaded fat chick thought, how will I know? It's kind of rare, after all, for the people you pass to point, sneer, or make gagging noises.

Of course, some days are easier than others. Some days the waistband of my Lycra shorts creates multiple rolls of fat around my midsection. Some days my sports bra feels like one side or the other is going to burst. Some days I seem to be moving so slowly that I'm bound to attract attention, the way the old dude in the fishing hat attracts attention by driving forty miles an hour on the freeway. Some days I feel so fat, old, and creaky that I just give up on the day's plans and watch a baseball game instead. But the secret is to keep those days to a bare minimum and plod onward with cheerful determination through all the other days. Usually after I've been out for twenty minutes or so, I'm not so aware of the waistband or the sports bra or even how slowly I'm moving. I'm just aware that I am moving, and it's good.

So whenever you pull on your workout clothes, even if they have spandex in them, remember that you deserve to be out there doing whatever it is you're going to do. If you're riding your bike, you have just as much right to be there as Lance Armstrong does. Your right to be in motion, your right to be athletic, your right to be strong and fit—these rights are inalienable. It's your life and it's your pursuit of happiness. Don't let anybody take that away from you.

THE LOWDOWN: MAKING THE WORDS REAL

How do you abandon self-consciousness? Isn't it ingrained into every fiber of our media-saturated, dissatisfied being? Well, yes, and shedding it takes time and practice. But this is how you start.

Embrace the fact that you are physically and mentally imperfect. Say it out loud. Maybe even write it down.

Accept that no matter how hard you work out, you are never going to have a "perfect" body. Say that out loud too: "I am imperfect and I will always be imperfect."

Celebrate the fact that being imperfect does not matter. Say something like, "Woo-hoo! I am free of the pressure of impossible striving for perfection!" or whatever your particular idiom moves you to say.

Identify an athletic goal that you want to achieve: ride a bike one hundred miles, hike to the top of the tallest mountain within a thousand miles, spike a volleyball, carve swooping turns on a snowboard. Say, out loud, that you can accomplish this feat even with big thighs or droopage in the upper arms. As for how to identify an athletic goal, if it isn't already living somewhere in your head or your guts, take a look at Chapter 7.

If you choose to run a marathon, repeat to yourself, out loud, every night and every morning, "I can and will run a marathon even if my thighs never get any smaller as a result of all my hard training."

Go do the things that will enable you to do your athletic thing. If you've always dreamed of playing tennis like Serena Williams, go sign up for classes again. Beginners' classes, if that's where you're at.

Hold your head high. Say to yourself, "I look okay, I feel great, and I don't give a crap what anyone else thinks." Practice during this, and eventually it will become second nature, on most days at least.

SEE FITNESS AS
WHAT YOU DO,
NOT HOW YOU LOOK

WHEN I WAS doing research for this book, I looked at other books about fitness. What I found, though, was not, in my definition, about fitness. The books were about looking good, with titles like *Look Awesome in the Buff*, *The Sacred Text of Body Sculpting for Women*, *Sculpt Your Way to Feminine Perfection*, and *Be a Babealicious Hottie in 20 Minutes a Day*. It was all about looking cute and "sculpting." I'm not trying to say that weight training is bad, far from it. But doing it so that you are perfectly "sculpted" or look great naked is ignoring the miracle of all the other stuff you can do with your body.

Sculpting is fine if you happen to be a piece of marble or a chunk of bronze. But you and I, girlfriend, are living, breathing, moving combinations of muscle and bone, ligaments, veins, arteries, organs, glands, and of course fat cells. And the operative word is "moving." Fitness comes from moving and is about moving. It's all about the ways you can utilize your incredible array of body parts to do things. Real things, not just endless repetitions on a quadriceps extension machine or a bench press. Don't get me wrong, I love bench presses. I love the gym, and I love strength training exercises. I even like those exercises for their own sake.

But a regimen that enforces sculpting and shaping as its primary goal has almost nothing to do with real fitness. Instead, it is slavery to a pervasive set of ideas that we buy into that we must strive for perfection in our appearance, perfection is something achievable, and looking great is our most important purpose. These books talk about strength, which is good. But they talk a lot about reduction of body fat. Much as we know we're supposed to get rid of body fat in order to be healthy, the real reason most people want to get rid of their body fat is to look good.

Go into any bookstore and you'll find a dozen tomes of this ilk, feeding a fantasy that you can look like one of these fitness models if you just work hard enough. They promote the idea of fitness as zero body fat, perfect proportions, and aesthetically pleasing amounts of muscle. The problem with this genre of fitness books is that their authors are not paying attention to what's really important: real-world movement and fun. What are you going to do with that body once you've sculpted it? Are you going to spend an hour and fifteen minutes in the gym five days a week, and the rest of your time admiring yourself in the mirror? Sure, you can admire your progress—for three or four minutes at most. Then what?

I invite you to consider fitness as a triumph of function. Function on the cellular level, on the level of individual muscles, but mostly on the level of what your whole body and mind can do together when you put your heart into whatever it is you do. Whether it's riding a bike for one hundred miles, learning to dance red-hot salsa, finishing a triathlon, kicking the heavy bag right off its hook, or hitting a dead straight drive onto the middle of the fairway, fitness is what you can do, not how you look.

Rebecca Bailey is a woman who was athletic just as women's sports were starting to blossom. She's a mom, a therapist, a volleyball player, an ex-discus thrower, and now a triathlete. She was lucky enough to understand from childhood that the point of sports was doing great things:

In junior high in 1973 there was only softball, gymnastics, and volleyball offered for girls. I was a strong, big-boned, wide-shouldered German girl, not built like the petite gymnasts. I played softball and volleyball. I was stronger than many, but certainly not the strongest member of the teams. In high school, I played volleyball, and I discovered track and field. I always secretly thought I could be a sprinter and wished someone would ask me to try. But the coach saw my muscular frame and my family history, and I never even got a chance to try to run. My sister and my stepbrother both held school track and field records in the discus, and my stepbrother patiently spent hours in the backyard teaching me the art of throwing. Suddenly my big bones and muscular frame were a real asset; I had a sport I really excelled in. I spent hours during the off-season working out in the weight room with the boys. I had great genetics for strong shoulders and muscular legs. I loved being big and strong before being muscular and fit was popular for women. The 1970s encouraged women to look like Twiggy, the first anorexic model. I thought she looked stupid. Why would I want to aspire to that? I was almost 5 feet 7 inches, and during my prime, I was a buff, lean, discus-throwing machine, weighing in at 170 pounds with less than 20 percent body fat. I broke my sister's discus throwing school record early in my junior year, and by my senior year I was one of the top five or ten female high school discus throwers in Washington State.

Function. Function over form, function triumphing over functionality to become poetry, to become beauty, to become art. And doesn't that sound like fun?

THE LOWDOWN: MAKING THE WORDS REAL

The tricky thing about some of the early parts of this fitness program is that the critical parts of the approach take place inside the labyrinths of your brain. But since you probably picked up this book to figure out what to do with your body, we'll compromise. I'll give you some brain stuff to work on while you move your body. Here are some ways to practice thinking differently about fitness and incorporating that thinking into your movement:

Notice other people doing cool athletic things, especially people who are similar in age, gender, body type, or other distinguishing characteristic. Make a point of appreciating the old geezer on the thirty-year-old steel-frame French road bike, the thick girl in the aerobics class, the final finisher in your local 5k race. Go to events to find these people if you don't see them around your neighborhood, because they are out there, doing their thing.

Appreciate those people. They are living the Way of the Imperfect Athlete. See how the thickset women do all the same moves as the thinner ones.

continues

The Lowdown: Making the Words Real *continued*

Notice the things your body can do now. Every time you get up off a low couch, you are achieving a small miracle of strength and coordination. (Try not to grunt as you get up—it detracts from the sense of the miraculous.) Go outside and take a walk around the block or put on the tunes that make you dance like you were sixteen again. While you're moving, notice things that you normally take for granted, like the balance that keeps you from falling down. This is not a "well, duh" but rather a finely tuned, incredibly complex interaction of systems. Notice how your feet, calves, knees, and thighs all work together to keep you moving, and how your arms naturally swing to balance your movement. This is the beauty of function, and this is what you build on to become an athlete.

There's a cliché in fitness writing that tells you to take the stairs instead of the elevator whenever you can. Yes, yes, it's true, though I'd much rather take the elevator. But when I do take the stairs, I make a point of thinking of it as strength training, and appreciating the work that my legs, back, hips, butt, and even abdominal muscles are doing to get me from the ground floor to the first floor. So take the stairs, even one floor, and take them as an athlete.

If you're already doing regular exercise, take time to think about what it really means to lift weights for twenty minutes or ride the equivalent of ten miles on an exercise bike. Go to Google maps and see how far ten miles is from your house. Do some math about the amount of weight you just lifted. Two sets of ten dumbbell curls with ten-pound weights on each arm is . . . um . . . four hundred pounds. That's a lot. And that's just one exercise for your upper arms.

BE SLOW

I AM AN expert on being slow. I wouldn't say I am the world's premier expert—there must be someone out there who is slower than I am, even at running—but I did write a whole book called *Slow Fat Triathlete*, so I must know something.

One thing I realized even before I sent the book out into the world is that the title contains two words that are frankly taboo in middle-class American culture. Number one on that list of course is the F-word. "Fat" is not a word that many Americans, especially women, use to describe themselves, unless it's in a self-deprecating oh-please-correct-me-because-I'm-not-really way, like "Oh my god, I'm so-o-o fat right now."

The other taboo word is "slow." We are not a society that values slow. We are into fast food (notoriously), interstate highways, Internet banking, and speed dating. If you're under twenty, e-mail is too slow; you have to text. Overnight delivery is too slow—just let me download it, okay? Americans value hitting the ground running, getting up to speed, steep learning curves, rapid acceleration, and just-in-time delivery. We go straight to the top; we pass GO as fast as we can. We do not, as a culture, place great value on moseying, lollygagging, or plodding.

But there I am, pretty slow. And, depending on my current ability to control my unnatural appetite for french fries and mayonnaise, I'm also pretty fat. Not surprisingly, these two qualities are correlated. The fatter I am, the slower I get.

Over the last couple years, as I regained big chunks of weight I had lost, I started to run more and more slowly. Where once I used to strive for sub–ten minute miles, I was creeping up to twelve-, thirteen-, and eventually fourteen-minute miles, while still trying as hard as I could. It was discouraging, but because I had written *Slow Fat Triathlete*, I couldn't give up simply because I felt I was too slow and too fat. When I wrote the book, I was still improving my times, still moving in the "correct" direction as an athlete. But I still told my readers, "Hey, it doesn't matter how slow you are. It only matters that you are out there participating." It sucks being forced to take your own advice. The only consolation is that I believe it. In terms of enjoying your exercise, your workout, or even your race, it really doesn't matter whether you're slow or fast.

When I went to Albany to do a speaking gig for a women's group, I stayed with a cheerful and wise woman named Mary Jane who had been training for months for the Pine Bush Triathlon and knew she was going to be slow. "Well," she said, "I look at it this way: triathlon is an endurance sport, so whoever comes in last wins at enduring the longest." And this is true. If you're out enjoying a beautiful morning in a scenic area, what's the rush? The slower you are, the more you get to enjoy the experience.

Some incipient triathletes write to me about their fears and insecurities. The number one fear is probably swimming in open water, and the number two fear is probably finishing last. I think to myself, wait a minute—you're more worried about finishing last than about, say, wiping out on the bike and suffering a traumatic brain injury? Or having a heart attack? If you finish last, *you finish!* You get to wear the race T-shirt, and nowhere on the shirt does it say "Last place! Slowest-ass athlete of the day!" You get the same finishers' medal as that wiry chick who smoked the field.

Danskin sponsors a fantastic series of triathlons for women all over the country, and if you're interested, you ought to check out the nearest Danskin tri. (Unless you're a guy, in which case, sorry. Drop me an e-mail and I'll find you the perfect first triathlon, I promise.) One of the things I like best about Danskin is that the final triathlete to cross the finish line is treated like a star. Sally Edwards, a grande dame of the sport, a hero to thousands of triathletes, breast cancer survivor, and gifted motivator, always crosses the line with the final finisher, hand in hand. That lucky finisher gets diamonds, luggage, massages, and other fabulous prizes, seriously! It's very moving to see everyone who is left at the race cheering wildly, celebrating the accomplishment of the woman who endured the longest. In her essential book, *Triathlon for Women*, Sally writes, "I prefer being the last to finish: It's the best place in the race for one reason—the vantage point of being behind tens of thousands of women competing in their first triathlon."

The principle of going slow and being happy about it can easily be applied to other athletic and fitness endeavors. Maybe you go to the gym and take a cardio kickboxing class but you don't throw those combo punches and kicks with the same snap as the girls in the front row with the well-defined abs and the low-rise shorts. That's okay. If you were actually going to step into the ring and spar, the speed of your reactions and punches would be an issue. But in a noncompetitive environment, go at your own pace.

Or say you are training for one of those three-day breast cancer walks and the group you train with walks faster than you do. It can be hard, but it's okay to just let them go ahead. Your pace right now is your pace. You can go a little faster than your natural pace for a while, but eventually you will need to drop back and recover. That's how you build fitness. You go slow, then you push a little, then you go slow again.

Opera singer, certified aerobics instructor, and personal trainer Jeanette de Patie is a firm believer in the power of slow. The creator and star of *The Fat Chick Works Out* fitness DVD is a marathoner and sometime triathlete who leads aerobics classes for people who fear a "regular" aerobics class would kill them. She encourages participants to go at their own pace and will even cut short the class for a chat session if she senses that anyone is struggling and feeling left behind.

Slow is good for strength training too. The latest research in human kinesiology (the study of how we move) indicates that if you do your biceps curl or your stomach crunch slowly, you'll gain more benefit than if you do it fast. You get more little muscle fibers working when you go slow. Slow is also good in yoga and is often required. The cool thing about yoga and slowness is that yoga also makes you slow your mind. One of the epidemic problems of our multitasking, overscheduled modern lives is that our minds are always racing. We're always thinking about what we need to do next. Yoga helps you focus on what you're doing now.

Focusing on the moment is to me one of the key benefits of exercising, and sometimes going slow is what it takes to achieve that focus. At least when you are going slow you can maintain that focus for longer. If I'm sprinting full out for one hundred yards, I'm completely focused on the moment, but the moment only lasts seventeen seconds or so (I told you I was slow). If I jog along for an hour at a placid pace, that's a whole hour I have to slow my thoughts down, think about my breathing and about how my feet are striking the ground, think about my heart beating and my arms swinging. I make a special point of smelling the roses in my neighbors' yards.

So go ahead and plod. Mosey. You don't need to stop and smell the roses, just slow down enough to catch a whiff as you trot by.

 ## HOW SLOW CAN YOU GO?

Next time you go out for exercise, make a point of slowing down, at least for the first fifteen minutes or so. Go slow enough that it seems embarrassing, and then slow down even more. How slow can you go and still increase your fitness? There are a few ways to estimate your exertion.

There's the "talk test." If you're going too slow or too easy, you should be able to sing while you're exercising. If you're exerting yourself moderately, you should be able to carry on a conversation. If you are breathing too hard to talk beyond grunts and "uh-huh," that is considered vigorous activity. If you use this scale, you should stay firmly in conversational mode for the first part of your exercise. If you're new to moving yourself about, you shouldn't push yourself much past that range for four to six weeks, depending on your age, prior experience, and medical history.

continues

How Slow Can You Go? *continued*

The Centers for Disease Control and Prevention encourage exercisers to use the Borg Rating of Perceived Exertion. (Resistance is futile.) The Borg Scale goes from 6 (on the couch) to 20 (something like sprinting to the finish of the Olympic marathon—insanely hard). The reason it doesn't go from 1 to 15 is that your Borg rating times ten would roughly correlate to heart rate (more later on that). If you dig the Borg, your warm-up and cool-down should stay in the 11 to 12 range.

While warming up and cooling down, there should be no feeling of suffering or struggle. You should feel like, "Hey, I can do this all day." In the middle part of your workout, you can always ramp up your intensity if you want to. But the slower you start, the more thoroughly your body will adapt when you go faster.

BE PROUD

"**S**AY IT LOUD:** I'm [blank] and I'm proud!" No, I don't mean that you are blank. Although if you want to be blank and proud, go right ahead. This book is all about feeling that who you are is okay. I mean for you to fill in that blank with the adjective that most impedes you from getting out and doing the things you dream of doing in the physical arena—or heck, even in the emotional, career, or spiritual arena. Are you too old? Are you too klutzy? Have you been injured too many times? Are you too fat? Too weak? Too slow? Do you think of yourself as too lazy or too undisciplined?

Go ahead, say it loud, "I'm klutzy and I'm proud!" Sounds weird, huh? I'm old and I'm proud? I'm fat and I'm proud? That's some weird-ass shit right there. We're not supposed to think of ourselves that way, are we? Here's how I interpret that phrasing. It's not so much that I'm proud to be fat, it's that I'm a fat person who is proud. I'm proud of who I am and what I can do, fat and all. I'm proud of what my body can do. This body carried me through a marathon, even with a head cold and blisters. It's carried all 247 pounds of my forty-five-year-old self up and down mountain passes over 11,000 feet. Sometimes, on my bad days, I'm not so proud. But I keep working so that I have more days of pride than otherwise.

And when I'm proud, it's like a layer of feather-light body armor against the stares and prejudices and thoughts that I imagine other people are directing at me. It takes me way beyond just not being self-conscious. It gives me the chutzpah to look the hyperlean club cyclist in the eye and say, "Nice day for a ride." It gives me the grace to smile at the large woman jogging toward me and know that she is my sister, not my evil image in the mirror, the one I want to avoid. Pride, or self-respect if you prefer, opens me up emotionally. I can empathize with all the other exercisers I see in the park. I feel like part of the community rather than an isolated loser on the fringe. I go from hoping no one notices me to going out of my way to make contact with my fellow imperfect athletes.

And every time you take yourself out for a session of exercise (or keep yourself in the house for a session of wild gyrating to "Solid Gold Disco Hits") you're laying another stone in your foundation of pride. You battled the forces of entropy and scored a victory. Can I hear a big ol' "woo-hoo!" from the congregation?

And don't just build your foundation of pride out of physical accomplishments. Look at all the other things you do that take determination, persistence, generosity of spirit, creativity, and resourcefulness. Whether you work a high-pressure job, give your utmost as a caring parent, volunteer to rescue abandoned kittens, create tasty and nutritious meals in thirty minutes or less, or all of the above, there are probably at least six ways in which you kick butt every single day. Make a point of enumerating them and then pointing out to yourself, "Well, if I can close that $2 million deal, surely I have the wherewithal to make myself take a brisk walk around the park." Darn tootin' you do!

Some days you may even be proud of the fact that you decided you were really tired and you needed to nestle into the couch under your down throw and take a nap instead of working out. Sometimes that can be a hard decision to make. You feel like you might lose all your momentum and your hard-won store of pride if you skip that day's planned exercise and become one with your sofa instead. But if you bank enough things that you can put into your foundation of pride, you'll know that you'll be back, recharged and full of energy.

Before long, you'll be putting things into your structure of pride that you never imagined you could do. I don't think Indigo Brude ever imagined she would ride her bike solo across the United States, or that Paula Stout planned to manage an expedition base camp on Mount Everest. These were just things that grew out of years of building on small accomplishments and then bigger ones.

Yeah, sure, it can be scary trying to be proud, and it can be tough. We're assaulted at every turn with messages that we're not doing enough. We're not making enough money, we're not saving enough for retirement, our houses aren't clean enough, we're not spending enough time with our children, we are not thin enough, our blood pressure is too high, we're not eating enough whole grains.

Fight back. Be proud anyway. Even if you have to pick something microscopically small to be proud of in your quest to be more physically active, do that small thing. And then go out, or stay in, and move around and be proud.

THE LOWDOWN: MAKING THE WORDS REAL

Anyone who undertakes a fitness initiative—whether it's to move more, have more fun while moving, get fit for a trek in Bhutan, or build enough stamina to dance all night at your high school reunion—will benefit from keeping a journal of some sort. Whether you do it in an Excel spreadsheet, use an online journaling tool, or write it on a yellow legal pad, it's fun and gratifying to track what you did, when you did it, how you felt when you did it. And one of the things it's good to put in your journal is something you're proud of on the day. You may be proud that you got all the way down on the floor during your pigeon pose. You may take pride in running for five minutes longer than you ever have before. You may take pride in the fact that you felt proud for the first time out in the park. Look back after a month of doing your thing and see how much you have to be proud of. You hiked four miles with fifteen pounds in your pack! You looked at yourself in the mirror and smiled, on two different days. Each grain of pride may seem minuscule by itself, but the key is to start piling up those grains until you're standing on a mountain.

EMBRACE THE AWESOME POWER OF FUN

A **LOT OF PEOPLE** don't exercise because they think it's not going to be fun. And maybe it never has been fun for them. Maybe the thought of exercise conjures up the sadistic spirit of that tenth grade gym teacher whose joy in life was watching pimply adolescents run until they begged for mercy. Perhaps it brings back tormenting memories of being hit in the face with the ball they could never catch. Maybe to them it seems boring and monotonous. It seems like work, not fun. That's how they define it to themselves, and in many ways, that's how the culture defines it. I mean, come on, it's a workout, right? Not a "fun out." Nobody ever calls up a friend to say, "Hey, I'm going to go play on the weight machines at the gym. Wanna come?" No, people "work out" with weights. Coaches never write on the white board, "Fun out for Tuesday, 8/22" with sets of running or swimming intervals, soccer drills or weight sets.

Even Lisa Engles, the stellar track coach for Silicon Valley Triathlon Club, who's infamous for working on club members to redefine unpleasantness as something, well, less unpleasant, doesn't give us fun outs. She tells us to tell ourselves, "I don't experience this as pain, it's just the sensation of training hard." But she doesn't write "fun out" on the white board. Although, I will admit, she does sometimes have us do some pretty fun sessions, mostly as the triathlon season winds down. Relay races, skipping drills, races to see who can be the fastest to do ten push-ups, turn around three times, and sprint barefoot across the grass to his or her running shoes without collapsing from dizziness and laughter.

Let's get serious about fun. Fun is not just frivolity and noodle salad. Fun is a matter of life and death. Well, okay, maybe not life and death per se, but certainly life as it is meant to be lived. Without fun you don't get to be your truest self. With fun, though, you get to feel the joy of the stuff you do every day. You also get to experience peak moments—times when you look around and say, "This is what it's all about, right here, right now." Finally, it means that you regularly get into a state of flow, or into the zone, or get unconscious, or maybe get fully conscious—into a state where the only important thing is what you're doing at the moment. There's no room for worry, for planning, for regret, criticism, or for anything except getting out of the way of what your body and mind are doing together.

Is fun compatible with a life of regularly scheduled activities that have the aim of making you a fit, possibly even athletic person? For many people, the pinnacle of fun involves a beach, a lounge chair, and a highly alcoholic umbrella drink. For many of those same people, fun does not involve any of the following: (1) having your own (or anyone else's) sweat run into your eyes due to exercise-related activities; (2) a burning, exhausted sensation in any major muscle group; (3) sitting around with ice packs on your knees, ankles, feet, or hips, "just as a precaution"; (d) getting so red in the face that Russians try to make borscht out of your head. For others, any or all of the above would be okay as long as they also involve sex.

Some people engage in sports that consist of actual games: basketball, tennis, softball, volleyball, whatever. For them the words "play" and "game" are intrinsic to the language of the sport. Other people do things for fun that involve movement, and sometimes even sweating, but that's not considered exercise as such. Dancing your butt off at a club is a great way to get in shape, but nobody thinks of it as a workout. Climbing up and down ladders, pruning trees, carting grass clippings off to the bin, digging up the earth, that sort of thing is not my idea of fun (in fact it's my idea of hard labor), but millions of people garden as a hobby, and you can work up a sweat doing that, for sure.

Endurance athletes have to apply imagination and energy to find the fun in their sports. Marathon training doesn't look much like fun to the outside world, though race day is often festive. Triathlon, I think, looks a little more fun. There's the profound silliness of putting on a wetsuit, engaging in a titanic struggle with something that makes you look either like an aquatic superhero or a total dork, or both. There's the glee of stumbling out of the water, dizzy from the cold water in your ears, only to jump straight onto a bicycle and pedal maniacally off down the road. But the training, the endless sessions of swimming up and down, up and down the same old pool, staring at the black line on the bottom; the butt-numbing hours on the bike; the thousands and thousands of steps along the neighborhood streets, or trails if you're lucky—how is that fun, exactly?

Well, let's step back for a minute and take a look at some other activities that are common to many humans. Food, for example. Eating is fun. Many cultures have elevated the simple act of consuming enough calories to stay alive into one long joyous celebration of color, texture, aroma, contrast, and harmony among flavors, and the communal roots of human society. Food is fun, but it doesn't have to be fun. We have to eat whether it's fun or not. If we don't eat, we die. It's that simple. But we have invested some of our considerable intellectual, creative, spiritual, and emotional resources into food as art or craft, and when we don't get that out of our food, we are the poorer for it. Sex is fun. And it doesn't necessarily have to be fun either, right? I mean, there are probably a bunch of evolutionary-biological-sociological hypotheses about this. For example, that pleasurable sexual relations create stronger pair bonding, thus contributing to the likelihood of success in raising offspring to maturity. That sort of thing. But the future of the species depends on mating, so if we don't do it, we die. Collectively, that is. It's imperative to survival, whether it's fun or not. Sleep? Extremely pleasurable. And once again, why do we enjoy it? We have to do it, or—all together now—we die. It could be just something that happens, that we're not normally aware of, like breathing.

So those are some pretty basic functions of survival—eating, coupling, sleeping—that are really quite fun. But what about movement? Movement is also necessary for survival. Picture our hunter-gatherer ancestors on the primeval plains. These folks needed to move. They needed to be able to jog after the antelope or bison for hours, if not days. They roamed far and wide in search of edible roots, grasses, seeds, grubs, what have you.

(With that menu, it's pretty astonishing that humans developed any enjoyment of food whatsoever, don't you think?) They also lifted heavy objects, animals, rocks, building materials, baskets full of tasty grubs. They squatted and got up, squatted and got up, ad infinitum, dozens or hundreds of times a day. Imagine our fate as a species without the ability to move and exert physical energy for extended periods. And every culture that I'm aware of developed celebrations of movement—dancing, games, contests of agility, endurance, and strength.

So, if movement, like food, sex, and rest, is vital to our essence, why has the pleasure gone out of it? Why do so few of us associate a fifty-mile jog on the trail of an impala with the same kind of pleasure that appertains to a five-course prix fixe meal at Le Mouton Noir with accompanying wines? Heck if I know.

People who hate exercise probably see physical effort as distinctly not fun. Effort sucks and should be avoided. This makes sense for people whose day jobs involve actual hard work. Why would more energy output be fun? But with our increasingly outsourced, automated, service-oriented economy, the percentage of people who work primarily with their bodies is declining. A lot of us spend most of our working lives sitting or standing.

But if you make yourself believe that effort is fun, the whole game changes. Instead of thinking of your run as minute after endless minute of persistent, mind-numbing effort, focus on something that makes it a game for you. Think of running as a dance, where you put your mind on making each motion, each part of each stride, as graceful and fluid as you can. Embrace the sweat. Accept breathing hard. Just as a thought experiment, reframe the sensations that you experience when your body is working harder. Just forget to think of it as uncomfortable.

Imagine yourself with the rest of your tribe, jogging after a herd of antelope as the sun sinks low in the west.

Lisa Engles agrees. Even though she coaches world-class triathletes, she encourages everyone to have fun: "I think it's important to change the linguistics around exercise. 'Exercise' has a negative connotation for many people, so why not do something that sounds different, like a 'movement adventure.'? Just changing the language around this whole idea of exercise can shift our perception of what it is and how it feels.

"Make up crazy silly names for your workouts. Don't even call them workouts. Call your runs 'linear pavement dances.' If it makes it feel more enjoyable and fun then that's what you need to do.

"If our belief is that exercise is that hard and tedious, then we're not going to do it. If our belief is that movement is easy and effortless, and provides us with all these great physical and emotional benefits, that belief will help us to transform how we are, not just what we do. And exercise is often something that we 'do'; fun is a way of being. It's easy to think to yourself, 'I love to be a fun person. I'm a fun person.'"

Exercise is a pleasure that deserves its rightful place in the pantheon of hedonism. I could make this idea into a public health pitch, a plea to redefine exercise as fun before we all keel over from heart disease and stroke. But what I really want is for people all over the world to feel the groove of movement, to get up and dance and shake your body and bubble with joy. Whether it's on the basketball court or in the weight room or the pool, on the roads or on the trails or the boxing gym, be loose, be free. Have fun. Please. When you're having fun, real fun, you're most in touch with your best self. If this still seems impossible, keep reading. We're going to be looking at specific skills for developing your perception of fun and brainwashing yourself into loving movement in the chapters ahead. We'll talk about flow, and affirmations, and singing to yourself as you exercise. Trust me, it'll be fun.

THE LOWDOWN: MAKING THE WORDS REAL

How can you make exercise fun, especially with that grumpy PE teacher looming in your memory?

Get social. Enlist a friend, take a class, join a club. A good class, whether dance, martial arts, spinning, or water aerobics, makes the whole event seem more like a party. Or get three friends to join you for "no excuses" walks, jogs, bike rides, or swims.

Put on the tunes. While I'm not convinced that all physical activity needs to be accompanied by an iPod, the beats and festive sounds of your favorite musical genres can bring an element of fun to the perceived discomfort of your exercise.

Be juvenile. Play with your kids, if you have them, or someone else's, if you can borrow them. Or play kids' games without any kids. Get out a hula hoop (now enjoying a fitness resurgence) or paddle ball set. Play Wii tennis or Dance Dance Revolution.

Sing while you exercise—or at least during the lower-intensity parts of your workout. Buy a pair of bright green socks and wear them.

Run backward. It's good for your knees and your balance. But make sure you do it on the straight part of a track or some similarly safe spot.

continues

The Lowdown: Making the Words Real *continued*

Wear a funny hat.

Talk to the person next to you on the treadmill.

Think of the ten funniest things that have ever happened to you.

Work a dance step into the middle of your run.

Find a deserted stretch of road or a parking lot and execute a series of swooping turns on your bike or your inline skates.

Picture yourself as a superhero. Imagine your bright gold and navy cape billowing splendidly behind you, even if you are on a stationary bike.

Laugh a lot, no matter what you're doing. If you fall down, trip over your feet, make the wrong move, hit the ball into the trees, whatever—make a point of giggling about it. If you see something cool, smile. No grim face.

START SMALL

AMBITION IS A laudable thing. Without it, Everest would not have been scaled; Columbus would not have sailed for the spicy enticements of the Indies; the mile would not have been run in under four minutes. To me, the very idea of a human being running a mile in under four minutes is still more astonishing than NASA's finest strolling on the moon.

What causes a lot of trouble for people who develop ambitions to move their bodies is that they think they can climb Everest right away or run the four-minute mile. They get all fired up, buy all the gear, and set out to conquer brave new worlds. Then they realize they're not pioneer miler Roger Bannister or prototype super-Kenyan runner Kip Keino, and they get discouraged. Or they get injured, and then they get discouraged. The gear sits in the garage or the closet, and the would-be athlete stays on the couch, declining steadily into an entropic state.

Fortunately, though, most of the time this kind of thing happens to people who are young and dumb. Sometimes to people who are old and dumb. But that wouldn't be you, right? It used to be me, for sure. When I was young and dumb I decided to train for a 10k run. I wanted to run it in a certain time, and I wanted to run it by a certain date. I hit both those goals, but I gave myself tendonitis in my foot that didn't go away for a couple of months. I got discouraged, retired to the couch, and started gaining weight, languishing for over a year.

Fitness author Suzanne Schlosberg agrees with me on this one: "If you suddenly make exercise your life's mission, you're going to burn out or get injured or both. I've seen it happen a zillion times. A friend discovers exercise, realizes how great it feels to sweat and to become fit, and then BAM—the honeymoon is over or they get hurt, and they never work out again. You've got to whet your appetite and leave yourself wanting more at the end of each workout."

If I had been as old and cautious and smart as I am now, I might have started small in my training. I might have decided to enter a 5k race before working my way up to the 10k. I would have increased my mileage gradually, and I wouldn't have pressured myself to go faster every time out. I would have started by scaling Charles Mound, the highest point in Illinois, at a dizzying 1,235 feet above sea level, before even looking at my Everest.

(Question: How flat does your state have to be when its highest point isn't Mount Something or even Something Hill, but Something Mound?)

Starting small is a vital component of being happily, shamelessly fit. There's no shame in walking one mile as the starting point for your three-day breast cancer walk. Nothing shameful about taking swimming lessons so you can do a triathlon.

I've heard people talk about their first triathlon in a self-deprecating tone, like, "Oh, it was only a mini tri." A mini tri? So the heck what? That was still something you had to train for, prepare for, and get up in the morning and actually accomplish at an hour when most of the good people of America are still sleeping and dreaming of their Sunday donuts. All right, if your shy and retiring personality requires that you belittle your own accomplishments in front of other people, go ahead. Demur, blush, disparage, but know in your heart that your small achievement is real, important, and big in ways that can't be measured by height or distance or time.

Bonnie Crawford from Portland started small. She was big at the time, but she started small. She weighed about 350 pounds when she joined Weight Watchers and Curves, and about thirty pounds less when she signed up for a 5k run/walk on New Year's Eve 2002. She struggled ahead of the final finishers—an elderly man pushing his wife in a wheelchair—but she got the bug.

"I sucked but I had finished and somewhere deep inside I knew I'd be back, I had to get better, to beat my time, to do more races. Clearly Curves was helping my stamina and cardio but it was not the same as walking, so I started walking once a week in addition to Curves. I got my fifty pounds lost magnet; I dropped below three hundred pounds."

Next Bonnie signed up for a sprint triathlon.

I was so nervous about swimming in a lake that I decided to sign up for a sprint triathlon relay two weeks before the Danskin triathlon. A friend of mine was going to run the 5k and I would do the swim and bike. I was so excited! I wasn't sure how I'd do, but I felt like I could finish and that was all that mattered. The relay day approached and I went to pick up my packet and T-shirt. I was bummed when I found out they didn't have XXL T-shirts. If I was doing the race I wanted to be able to wear the T-shirt. The race director looked at me and said, "I don't know any triathletes who need an XXL." Bingo, the gauntlet was thrown down, and I knew that I was going to prove her wrong. They found an XXL T-shirt that was meant for a volunteer and I finished the relay and got ready for my first triathlon.

Bonnie finished her first complete triathlon (where they did have size XXL shirts) and moved on to hundred-mile bike rides, a half marathon, and longer triathlons. In 2005, though, her progress was stalled by knee surgery and a subsequent blood clot. Undeterred, she rehabbed diligently and she returned to triathlon that same year.

Small is big. And big is cool.

THE LOWDOWN: MAKING THE WORDS REAL

There's nothing wrong with walking around the block as your first step. Even if it's a short block. So pick a tiny goal to start with. Jog and walk for twenty minutes. Get your decrepit old bike cleaned and tuned up. Once it's shiny and the gears shift cleanly, you probably won't be able to resist taking it out for a spin, but make it a short, easy one. Quit for the day well before your rump exhibits the first signs of rawness. Make it so you can't wait to get back on that bike the next day.

Or hey, do one push-up. Two days later set your goal for two push-ups. Then work it up to five. Then ten. Then twenty. Achieving little goals is fun. Then you can set another little goal. Break your massive mountain of ambition down into little nugget goals that you can pick up and toss into your bucket one at a time. And add every nugget into your journal of pride, along with the grains of pride sand that are already there. Each one represents accomplishment.

DREAM BIG

YEAH, **SURE, YOU** ought to start small. Begin with that first walk around the block or the first (yet somehow strangely difficult) push-up. You may be humbled by your early efforts, but I implore you, do not let the Lilliputian scale of those efforts limit the scope of your dreams. I am constantly amazed by the capacity of the bodies and minds of so-called average people to achieve exceptional things. And you are one of those people.

If you want to climb Everest, if you really truly do in your deep secret dreaming heart, don't be discouraged by the fact that your first assault on Charles Mound left you hobbled for days with cramping quads and tender calves. Don't be discouraged if you don't know what your quads are. You can learn. And you can get stronger. And you can, with patience and determination and the persistence of a pit bull, get up Charles Mound, and then Mount Sunflower in Kansas (which, science has shown, is flatter than a pancake), and then Mount Whitney, tallest mountain in the continental United States. You can learn how to hike with balance; how to strap on your pack to keep the load off your lumbar spine; how to use hiking poles and then an ice ax and crampons. If you progress further in your mountaineering career than I have, you may even learn to use the word "crampons" without snickering. Crampons. Hehe.

Everest, though, is not my personal dream. It's cold and scary and massively expensive, and your lips get chapped all to hell at 29,000 feet. When Paula Stout found herself in between high-paying corporate management jobs, she decided to use the time to go to Everest and become base camp manager for the Climbing for a Cure Everest expedition in 2005, a climb to raise awareness and funds to combat cancer. Base camp management was not something she had experience with, but Paula is a person who can dream big. Sure, she could organize a herd of cats to march in formation to the tune of "Funkytown," but coordinate the life-or-death logistics of high-altitude mountaineering? Wow! She had climbed some mountains in California, but California is a long way from Nepal. Paula never had to go higher on Everest than 18,000 feet or so, but in my view that is still plenty cold, scary, and lip-chapping. It's a big, big dream.

My dream is to ride my bike up the classic climbs of the Tour de France: the Alpe d'Huez, the Col du Galibier, the Col de Télégraphe. It's a fairly modest dream, athletically speaking. People do it every year, thousands of people. People I know have done it. And it's actually only one of my dreams. I want to finish an Ironman within the legal time limit and also, someday, do a pull-up. At the moment I'm working on the cycling dream. For me, it's a really big dream. It would involve climbs of, say, twelve miles—constantly going uphill. And then doing it again. And I am a cyclist who gets winded going up the little hill under I-280 on Foothill Expressway.

You may say that I'm not really starting small here because I've already been cycling for about five years, and I have done some rides of over fifty miles. I've even grunted my way up some of the local cyclists' "real" climbs, multimile grunt fests like Old La Honda Road and Kings Mountain, narrow, serpentine country lanes that start off in sunshine and manzanita and end up in redwoods and fog, what seems like thousands of feet higher. But besides weight gain and concomitant slowness, I suffered a bout of acute tendonitis in my wrist, which kept me off the bike for a couple of months. When I finally got back on my trusty steed, I had fallen to the level of my early training for my first triathlon. The gently rolling seven miles up Foothill to Page Mill Road and back were all I could handle.

But I have a plan. My plan started, as so many plans do, with whipping out a credit card, in this case for the purchase of a sparkling new bicycle. I didn't have the gear ratios to train for my dream. With the triple chainring on my LeMond Zurich, though, I'm ready to rock. So here's my plan. I gradually increase the mileage of my long rides each month. In April I push it up to eighty-five miles and multiple climbs. And by April 30 I make it through the Chico Wildflower Century, a hundred-mile epic around the hills and plains of a quaint almond-growing and university town. The Wildflower was selected for its tradition, its excellent food stops, its attractive jersey, and the good company. I know it has like 90,000 vertical feet of climbing (well, maybe more like 5,000), but I'm game for that. It's just like an endless series of leg presses. Plus I can stop every couple of hours for a great snack.

So that's phase one. I have to build up endurance in a lot of areas. First, my behind has to get used to being on a bike for six to eight hours at a time. This is facilitated partly, but not entirely, by the liberal application of a variety of unguents to the affected portions of the anatomy. (For more on chafing, see Chapter 22.)

I also have to accustom my body to work at a moderate to moderately hard pace for hours on end. This, like the booty conditioning, we do by gradually increasing the length of the long ride. We also carry lots of snacks in the back pockets of our bike jersey so we don't run out of blood sugar and bonk way out on the back roads, miles from a 7–11.

But the hardest thing is to learn to climb again. The quickest and most reliable way for me to become a better climber would be to lose a bunch of weight. And I will. Starting after the new year, of course. But I am not going to shy away from the hills until I lose the weight. I will just work on the shorter hills for a while, then work back up to the longer ones, even if I'm still fatter than I want to be as an aspiring conqueror of the Tourmalet. I will not let my excess weight keep me from aspiring to my lofty goal.

In phase two—after Wildflower Century—I will ride all the climbs that my area has to offer. Tunitas Creek, Saratoga Gap, even the 4,300 feet up Mount Hamilton and the desperately steep section of Hicks Road past the reservoir. I will ride those climbs until they don't scare me anymore. This will take me another year or so. And then, the following year, I round up a couple of crazy cycling buddies and we buy a ticket to France, and then my Big Dream will be real.

Oh, and what about Bonnie's dreams, Bonnie of the 350 pounds and the size XXL triathlon T-shirt? She finished her Ironman triathlon debut for Ironman Coeur d'Alene, Idaho, in July 2007, having lost 155 pounds and becoming a USA Today Weight Loss Challenge profile. Bonnie started small and ended up dreaming large. Extra, extra large. And so can you.

If you're still searching for your activity of choice, maybe the best way to find it is to go back to your childhood fantasies.

Were you a ninja, stealthy and silent? Try some martial arts. A mountain climber on the hill behind the house? Sign up with a hiking club or a climbing gym. A tightrope walker on the back fence? There are, in some places, companies that will teach you the circus arts. Take your fantasies, connect them to your adult life, and make a dream you can reach. Then make a plan.

BIG DREAMS FOR GOOD CAUSES: ATHLETIC ENDEAVORS FOR CHARITY

One tried-and-true way to keep yourself on the path of your Big Dream is to do it for a cause greater than yourself, whether it's leukemia and lymphoma, diabetes, challenged athletes, or breast cancer research. One of my first big athletic challenges was the March of Dimes Walkathon when I was in fifth grade. There was no way I could have walked twenty miles without a strong need to do something for a good cause and follow through on my commitment to my sponsors.

These days there are a zillion ways of being athletic for a good cause. Not all of them are as challenging as managing Everest base camp, either. If your sporting dreams would go better with charity, here are some options:

Team in Training (TNT). A massive organization that has trained over 300,000 people to do triathlons, marathons, half marathons, and century bike rides. TNT participants raise a boatload of money ($700 million and counting) for the Leukemia and Lymphoma Society, and in return they get coaching, group support, travel and lodging expenses, and the chance to participate in some very cool events with a crew of like-minded fellow athletes. Extremely supportive of everyone in the team, especially raw beginners.

continues

Big Dreams for Good Causes: Athletic Endeavors for Charity *continued*

Walk for Breast Cancer.   A series of two-day walking events to raise money for breast cancer research, screening, treatment, and support. Participants walk 26.2 or 39.3 miles over a weekend in cities across the United States. The event includes a Saturday night in a tent village set up by hundreds of eager volunteers. Great for women or for men who want to meet thousands of women in (walk.avonfoundation.org).

MS Bike Ride.   The National Multiple Sclerosis Society's local chapters produce rides, often 150 miles over two days, that together make up the largest charity ride in the country. You raise money, and the MS chapter helps you on your way. www.nationalmssociety.org.

Do-It-Yourself Fund-Raising.   You can become your own activist, using any event that you sponsor to raise funds for any cause you designate. The useful website *www.active.com* allows you to start a fund-raising page and collect donations online (in return for a small percentage that Active collects on each donation).

  There are also rides, runs, walks, and triathlons to benefit AIDS charities, ALS, diabetes, the American Heart Association, the American Stroke Association, or pretty much any condition or illness that speaks to your heart and soul. Get on Google. Get busy.

DON'T HATE

HATE IS A powerful emotion. I try not to indulge in it very often unless I'm talking sports. I hate the Yankees, the Dodgers, and the Dallas Cowboys, and I hate the Lakers with an unreasoning passion that has lasted for thirty-two years so far. I let myself do this because it's not real to me. The teams and players, coaches and general managers are just characters in my favorite soap operas. But what do I hate in the real world? What do you hate?

If you're a woman who is an aspiring imperfect athlete, chances are you hate your body. Or at least some parts of it. You've probably had some pet hates since you were a child, or at least an adolescent. I've hated my belly since I was probably eight or nine, and sadly, I began to hate my breasts just about as soon as they appeared, which was absurdly early for that bygone era. Girls are reaching puberty earlier now for some reason (hormones in their food? higher calorie intake? high-tech rays emitted by the spaceships of silver-skinned aliens who really, really like boobies?), but at the time it was pretty absurd to need a bra at age eleven. As my boobs expanded like jellyfish on steroids, I began to hate them more and more. They got in the way of everything, and I'm talking physically, not psychologically. They bounced, they wobbled, they spilled out of my always too small bras.

I came to hate bras with a passion previously reserved for the L.A. Lakers. The straps cutting cruelly into my shoulders, the band digging into my back and chest, the undignified wrestling match to get the damn thing on and off (my shoulders have never been flexible, so doing anything behind my back is like a torture devised by the Inquisition).

So, what do you hate? Your bulging thighs? Your thick ankles? Your knock knees? Your flat feet, pigeon toes, bowlegs, love handles, muffin top, flat boobs, giant boobs, flabby upper arms, bony hands, skinny calves, ghetto booty, or any combination of the above?

For most of the women I know, the hating is tied in with fat. I have known some folks who hated their skinny limbs, their overly white skin, their funny-shaped feet. But to me, nothing matches the raw hatred that fat induces. Some of the following quotes come from my interactions in the online world, where people are often more willing to let you know what really hurts:

"I've had more than my share of the 'oh you'd be so pretty if you were thin' comments. A family friend told me I would never get into an Ivy League school because I was fat (as if they ask for your weight on applications). And similarly, a cousin of my mother's called me one afternoon to tell me I would never succeed at any profession if I was heavy."

"When I was heavy, I was a 'nobody' to those around me. I was belittled by my family, my husband's family, and even well-meaning friends. I can't tell you the number of times I received clothes as a gift and was then told 'well, you can take it back if it doesn't fit—it looks like it might not.' The hurt fueled my poor eating.

"Until I remarried (became more sedentary) and quit smoking (replaced one hand-to-mouth activity with another), that is. Between those two events, I put on one hundred pounds. Whoa! Who *is* that woman in the mirror? That simply *cannot* be me!? I had always prided myself on being thin (even though I didn't realize I wasn't fit) even into my thirties, so to 'suddenly' become large was more than a little unsettling. . . . I was filled with self-loathing. I wasn't sexy anymore. I was a fat slob. I started wearing baggy clothes in an effort to hide the mounds of flesh that were collecting on my body. Everything jiggled. I couldn't roll over in bed without it being a two-part process. I hated myself, but felt powerless to stop it."

This is probably familiar stuff to you. If you get almost any group of female friends together for more than an hour, you will almost inevitably hear an interweaving conversation about the hated body parts, a jazz combo of almost improvisational genius, the high horns spiraling upward: "My arms are disgusting; my arms are disgusting," the alto sax wailing, "My stomach bulges over every pair of pants I own, whoa whoa whoa aaaaaaaaaaawhooooooooooooo," and the bass walking through, "My ass is huge; my ass is huge." It's an art form. We laugh, we share our insecurities, we release tension. But do we really need to do it?

What if we got together and tried a different set of themes and variations? What if we talked about how our thighs are powerful? How our backs are strong? Our ankles stable and not prone to spraining? Or what if we quit talking about our body parts altogether, even to ourselves? What if you or I got up in the morning and looked ourselves squarely in the eye in the foggy bathroom mirror and said, "Hey, this body works ok, and I'm grateful for it." Would that be hard? Yup. I was doing some indoor cycling at the YMCA last night, since it was dark and cold outside. To my consternation, the considerate YMCA staff had placed the spinning bikes right in front of the floor-to-ceiling mirror. I was pedaling away, trying to keep my posture relaxed, my cadence steady, and my core engaged and strong, when I looked in the mirror and observed that my reflection was roughly the dimensions of an adolescent hippopotamus. My first reaction was to avert my eyes from the sight. But then I said to myself, "No! That is not cool!" I looked back up, looked myself right in the eyes, and smiled at myself.

My fellow YMCA members may have thought I was a loony, but more likely they were not bothering to look at me or think about me at all. (See Chapter 1 for a refresher course on that.) I sure hope they weren't looking at me too hard, because as I observed myself, determinedly thinking positive thoughts about my body, I suddenly noticed that I had put on my bike shorts inside out, with the black fleece chamois pad around my crotch area hanging out there in the open for all to see. It could have been a lot worse. The shorts could have been bright gold or orange instead of a discreet dark blue. I kept pedaling, working hard to exude confidence and savoir faire. "This is how all the coolest athletes are wearing their shorts this winter" I projected to those around me. It totally worked. Trust me.

The other thing about the Y, or any other place where you exercise in close proximity to other people, is that it offers you lots of opportunities to hate those other people for the things that are right about their bodies and wrong with yours. This is just another way of hating your own body, so cut it out. Conversely, you can spend time focusing on the flaws of other people's bodies, workout outfits, and sweat volume. But, with all due respect, I sternly forbid you to engage in that sort of activity. It's not nice, and it feeds your paranoia that other people are thinking the same kinds of things about you.

Imperfect athletes need to spread joy and compassion, recognizing that everyone is struggling with self-hatred and insecurity. As we forgive others their flabby butts and bulging guts, we simultaneously forgive our own. So don't hate.

A final word from a Weight Watchers tri friend who is a two-time Ironman finisher: "These days, I'm no longer as heavy as I was, but I'm not as thin as I once was either. Fortunately the self-loathing has stopped. Becoming an endurance athlete has given me a new focus and a new source of pride. I may not be as thin as some of my contemporaries, but I can swim, bike, and run circles around them! I still want to be as thin as I used to be, but I would rather be at this fitness level and be that thin. If I can't have both, then I'll stay the size I am and that will be OKAY!"

THE LOWDOWN: MAKING THE WORDS REAL

For ten minutes every day for at least a month, and/or any time you catch yourself hating your [fill in your most hated body part here], stop and say, "This body works pretty well, and I'm okay with that." Say it out loud if you can, or whisper it to yourself, or say it mentally, but loudly.

You'll be a better athlete for it, and a happier and more popular person.

FIND YOUR INNER JOCK

YOU PROBABLY PICKED up this book because you aspire to be an athlete at some level. And because you're looking for a book to guide you, you may not have a clear vision of your inner jock.

Most people think of a certain type of person when they hear the word "jock." At my high school, that type of person was mostly a tallish, broad-shouldered young man with blond hair, a somewhat vacant stare, and a letterman's jacket. (My high school was not particularly multicultural.) Jocks were born to be athletes. They moved with grace, ran like young wolves, and looked effortlessly good in whatever uniform was in season. Nerdy boys like the ones I hung out with looked at them and felt inadequate.

As time passed and gender equity came to sports (thanks to Title IX), the girl jock came to prominence. Less broad-shouldered, perhaps, and less predictably blond, but lean and graceful, fast and strong, leveraging their physical gifts, their self-discipline, and their patiently honed skills into college scholarships in sports like basketball, soccer, softball, volleyball—not just traditional "girlie" sports like tennis and gymnastics. We saw the rise of Sheryl Swoopes, Bonnie Blair, Picabo Street, Paula Newby-Fraser, Hannah Teter. Now nerdy girls and fat girls and uncoordinated girls had other things to feel inadequate about besides their looks.

So what percentage of people are naturally superior athletes? Take your pick. Maybe 1 percent? How many are world-class, elite athletes like Venus Williams, Annika Sorenstam, Jackie Joyner-Kersee? Maybe 1/1000th of 1 percent? If there are 6.5 billion people on the planet, that means that only 65,000 of them get to be elite athletes, with almost half of them in India and China. Only about 3,000 are in the United States. So where does that leave the other 299,997,000 of us? Do we not get to be athletes because we'll never be elite? Uh-uh. No way am I buying into that.

We all get to be athletes if we want to, are willing to declare it, and are willing to put in sustained physical and mental work to reach our stated goal. We don't get to choose whether we have the freaky genes to actually win competitions with our speed or strength or agility, but we do get to choose whether we act like athletes, see ourselves as athletes, and treat ourselves like athletes.

The first step to becoming an athlete is determining your strengths. I use the word "strengths" loosely. I don't mean finding the things that will enable you to win a competition. Hey, let's keep the bar low here. I ain't about winning no competitions. (Though if I happen to do so, or even place third in the over-forty Athena division of a 180-person race, I'm just as delighted as the next person. Maybe even more so.) Figure out what your own strengths are and celebrate them, even if they are not traditional athletic advantages. Traditional athletic advantages would be attributes like speed, power, coordination, leaping ability, and so on.

At the end of this chapter you're going to take a look at the traits that will enable you to achieve your athletic dreams, both physical and mental. And your mental traits are going to be even more important to your success than the physical. Face it: if you'd been born with outstanding physical skills, you'd probably already think of yourself as an athlete. Or perhaps you were born with the ability to jump like Dwyane Wade and run like an antelope, and you've been slacking for a long time. Either way, you're going to need all the mental skills you can bring to bear on making yourself into a jock.

Take an inventory of your mental self. Did you go to work every day last winter even with a rotten case of the flu? If so, you could say, "I persevere even when I don't feel like it." Or else, "My employer has a crappy sick leave policy." Did you plan your best friend's wedding and never break a sweat? Then you are cool under pressure. Do you juggle soccer practices, work, school, kitchen duties, and cleaning up doggy barf? Then you are creative and resourceful at solving complex problems.

Why will you do this exercise? Because strengths are transferable. The same guts and talent for hard work that got you through night school plus a full-time job or through your summer job stacking cartons at the warehouse will get you through your marathon. You're giving the same sense of importance to your athletic endeavors that you did to earning your degree or your year's tuition or your kids' education. Whatever your goal is—learning to swim or doing the marathon or hiking the Appalachian Trail—you have to care about it that much. And you have to believe you have what it takes to make it happen.

So make a list of everything that makes you a potential athlete. And hold on to that list because you're going to need it.

THE LOWDOWN: MAKING THE WORDS REAL

What does being an athlete mean to you? What do athletes do every day? How do you approach exercise if you're an athlete? What do you think about your body? How do you treat it? What traits do you have in common with people you think of as athletes? You may not be particularly strong or fast, or quick with your hands or feet, but:

> You may be determined and persistent.
> You may be good at planning a project.
> You may be patient, willing to take the long view. You may be good at figuring out how to help people heal—knowledge that you can apply to your newly athletic self.
> You may be good at enduring.
> You may be compassionate. You may be good at seeing the funny side of your chosen athletic activities.

Take out your paper and pen, or your laptop and trackpad, and list at least ten characteristics that you have and how they are going to help you become an athlete. These attributes can be physical, mental, emotional, spiritual, or even financial. If you have the money to hire a personal trainer, for example, that's going to give you a leg up on your goals. But concentrate first on your inner resources. Think hard if you have to. Maybe you think you have no physical strengths. But dig deep. They're there. Have you ever had a sore back? No? Then write down, "I have a strong back." If you have managed to live to the age of, say, thirty-five without ever falling out of your heels (this one applies primarily, though not exclusively, to my female readers), write, "I have stable ankles." These are important characteristics for a beginning athlete. List at least three physical talents. Be creative. Two of my strengths

continues

The Lowdown: Making the Words Real *continued*

in triathlon are an ample layer of body fat that keeps me warm in cold water and helps me float, and weight that enables me to bomb down hills on a bike, unimpeded by the wind resistance that slows down lighter cyclists. You have strengths too. Write them down.

If you haven't yet figured out how to choose an activity that's right for you, use this exercise to help guide you. If you can tolerate cold water, you may want to look into the open water swim club. If you were a pretty good roller skater as a kid, you may want to take up roller hockey now. If you had great times on a bike, well, enough said.

SECTION II

TEN WAYS OF BEING AN ATHLETE

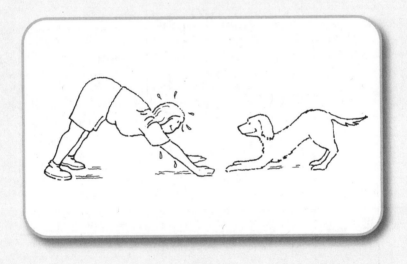

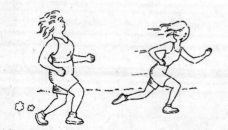

10

DARE TO WEAR LYCRA

DURING A TALK I gave on the promotional megatour for *Slow Fat Triathlete*, my guide to multisport fun for people of all shapes, sizes, and experience levels, the audience and I got into a discussion about what it's like to be out there wearing spandex. We were having a lively chat about self-consciousness versus the ability to go outside in bike shorts and not give a hoot about who sees you. Kelly, a teacher and a mom cruising through her forties with ample hips and thighs, told us of a recent cycling adventure on Martha's Vineyard. She had been riding a stationary bike throughout the winter and had just gotten a real bike when some friends invited her to ride the Vineyard with them. They were planning a fifty-mile ride, which is pretty ambitious for someone who just got her bike, but the friends said that Kelly could cut the ride short whenever she needed to.

Thus encouraged, Kelly packed her bike and headed for the ferry. She had real bike shorts—spandex/nylon bike shorts with padding (or chamois, as we call it in the Tour de France), but she was planning to ride in a long, baggy T-shirt. Kelly's friends convinced her that the baggy T-shirt would slow her down in the island's stiff sea breezes, as well as get sweaty and heavy as the day wore on. They offered her a spandex/nylon bike jersey but she resisted strenuously. No way would she be seen in public without something covering up her stomach, her butt, and her hips. Eventually the friends prevailed, and Kelly put on a bike jersey for the first time.

The early summer day was warm and bright. The cyclists meandered around the scenic back roads of Martha's Vineyard, stopping here and there for photographs, snacks, and drinks at local stores and cafés. As the day wore on, Kelly realized that she was feeling strong and would be able to ride the full fifty miles. This was an incredible accomplishment for someone who was for all intents and purposes doing her first real bike ride. But what amazed Kelly even more was that she was able to go into the stores and the cafés all exposed and "out there" in her spandex. It was really hard for her at first; she felt practically naked. But by the end of the day, it was something that felt pretty much fine. And that accomplishment—having the courage to go out in public as a larger woman wearing spandex—is what made Kelly choke up as she told her story. And she was not the only one.

I realize I've already spent time talking about how you need to let go of your self-consciousness and how you need to focus on all the great things your body can do rather than how your body looks while you're exercising or resting. But I think that the issue of form-fitting fabrics is worthy of its own bout of sisterly bonding. For many of us, even if we dare to go out in public and exercise, the question of what to wear can derail our best intentions. Since I have written *Slow Fat Triathlete*, I can't even tell you the number of e-mails I've gotten from readers who can't figure out what to wear for their first triathlon. A rather typical lament would be something like this: "I've tried on those triathlon outfits but I don't wanna look like a sausage covered in Lycra—what can I do? Please help!"

I sympathize: I also look like a sausage in my triathlon outfit. An extremely gaudy, red, white, and blue sausage with tan bits sticking out the sleeves and leg holes. No doubt about it, spandex reveals pretty much every imperfection.

Now let's review Chapters 1–2 for a few minutes. The first thing we do is abandon self-consciousness because we all have imperfect bodies and imperfections are really not a big deal. Next thing, we base our philosophy of fitness on preferring function to form. Fitness is about moving, not about sitting still and looking good. (I know that Chapters 1–2 were not that long ago, but if you're like me, you might read this book in chunks of three or four pages before you sink gratefully into an exhausted slumber at the end of every day.)

So if we accept the premises of Chapters 1–2, we realize that we have no reason to fear spandex, as it is generically known in the United States, or Lycra (trademarked by the company Invista, which used to be part of DuPont). Indeed, in a great number of diverse athletic pursuits, spandex is our friend. Repeat after me: "Spandex is my friend; I like spandex." Spandex is an eminently functional material, especially when combined with other useful materials like nylon and polyester.

Here's what Wikipedia, every lazy writer's number one research source, says about spandex:

> Spun from a block copolymer, these fibers exploit the high crystallinity and hardness of polyurethane segments, yet remain "rubbery" due to alternating segments of polyethylene glycol. This means that spandex can be stretched over 500% without

breaking; can be stretched repetitively and still recover original length; is lightweight and resistant to abrasion, body oils, perspiration, lotions and detergents; and is stronger and more durable than rubber. It is devoid of static or pilling problems.

It's also "soft, smooth, and supple."

I think we can all see how these properties benefit us as emerging athletes. Stretchiness is a valuable attribute for something that's going to cover your body when it moves. And of course we want the body to move. A lot. In lots of directions. We want the fabric to be lightweight, certainly, and abrasion resistance is also handy, especially when you have large thighs that tend to chafe against each other.

Wikipedia says that spandex has "poor strength," but hey, at least it's more durable and stronger than rubber. Which is good, because I have no interest in exercising in rubber shorts. And who can resist the fact that spandex is "soft, smooth, and supple"? I like that very much. And to top it all, spandex is even resistant to all of our natural yet somehow strangely soiling secretions, our artificial emoluments, and the detergents we use to clean them off.

Repeat after me once more: "Spandex is my friend."

Far from being uncomfortable in spandex-blend clothing, I actually find it soothing because you don't have to think about how it feels. It's the tactile equivalent of being invisible. It's just there, letting you do the things that you're out there to do—ride your bike, run around the park, skate along the river, climb the tree, whatever.

When I say "spandex" or "Lycra," I'm using these terms as a shorthand for form-fitting exercise clothing, not the slinky little black top you might wear clubbing or the Capri pants with that little extra bit of stretch. And as I mentioned earlier, spandex needs to be combined with other fibers in order to make useful exercise wear. In the fitness industry, the gurus of fabric design have come up with a number of useful (and sometimes pricey) materials grouped under the generic term "technical fabrics." There are names like Supplex and Tactel, Gore-Tex and DriFit, CoolMax and Climalite, most of which combine well with spandex. Almost everything benefits from a little stretch. The basic idea of most technical fabrics is that they help keep you dry when you're sweating. The little fibers transport moisture from your skin out through the fabric and into the outside air, where it magically goes away. The companies throw around terms like "ventilation channels" and "densely constructed polyester microfiber," but basically the idea is to keep you cool, keep you dry, keep you comfortable, and avoid chafing. (Chafing is not your friend.)

"But," I hear you say, "I don't think spandex is comfortable at all. I break out in hives and start to hyperventilate at the very thought of wearing spandex in public." I understand. I really do. So if you really need to wear that baggy cotton T-shirt and baggy cotton shorts to exercise, you should feel free. And if those fabrics work for you, great! But at some point you may find that your exercise is becoming more strenuous or taking more time, and that the cotton isn't standing up well to all the hard work—it's getting heavy and soaked with sweat, or it's bunching up in uncomfortable places, or it flops around, or, and this is the worst, it chafes. At that point, you might want to consider Lycra.

So let us salute Kelly's bravery in the face of years of self-consciousness, self-doubt, and even, and I don't think this is too strong a word, self-loathing. Let us grab our spandex bike shorts and wave them high in the air, banners of freedom and confidence, the hallmark of our liberation. But let's not forget to pull them over our butts before we go out on the bike ride. No sense in frightening the children too much.

THE LOWDOWN: MAKING THE WORDS REAL

How do we overcome our fear of spandex? Psychotherapists recommend creating a hierarchy of actions relating to a fear. For a person with a snake phobia, the hierarchy might start at the lowest anxiety level of reading about snakes, working up to looking at a live snake in a cage, and culminating with touching a live snake. So, making a reasonable analogy:

1. Go to the store and look at spandex workout clothes. Picture yourself in them. Picture yourself feeling strong, confident, and comfortable. Picture 10,000 people cheering you in your spandex as you accomplish your wildest athletic dream.
2. Buy some spandex. In your size. You don't have to wear it. Yet. Just have it around the house. Look at it. Touch it. Admire how soft, smooth, and supple it is. This process may take weeks, months, or even years.
3. Put the spandex on in the privacy of your own home. Jump up and down a bit. Jog a few steps. Wait until the house is empty if this makes you nervous. Look in the mirror and say, "I look totally fine. I deserve to wear this in public. I feel comfortable in these clothes."
4. Wear the spandex outside. Do it after dark if you have to.
5. Wear the spandex outside, in the daylight.
6. Enjoy.

OUTFIT YOURSELF JUDICIOUSLY

COTTON IS NOT the workout material of choice. It gets wet, it gets heavy, it can chafe and cause blisters. So what should you be wearing on your way to glorious, shameless fitness? Well, don't make too big a deal out of it. Some people have to have the right gadgets and clothes and equipment before they can be "real" athletes. Aspiring cyclists drop $5,000 on a full-carbon road bike, $250 on Italian cycling shoes, $130 on the helmet, and another $200 on the full set of Lance Armstrong Discovery Channel cycling duds. Only then do they feel prepared to tackle their goal. But just as you're going to start with what you already have in your physical arsenal, you can start with what you have in your closet or your garage, in many cases. We can't all work at Google and cash in our stock options to buy sporting goods, so we have to figure out what's essential and what's just for fun.

There is one area in which I will not skimp, and I will not let you skimp either: your footwear. Anything that touches your feet needs to be quality stuff. No matter what your sport is, take really good care of your feet. I guess if you're going to be spending most of your time in the pool, your shoes and socks don't need to have the highest priority, though you may want to invest in a quality pair of flip-flops. But any sport or activity that requires shoes also requires you to put the shoes at the top of your list.

I'm not just saying this because I'm a shoe-crazy girl jock. (I have only five active pairs of sport-related shoes, which is modest in the extreme for someone who does multiple sports.) I'm saying it because your feet are the foundation for everything you're going to be doing, whether it's running, walking, hiking, kickboxing, volleyball, or Ultimate Frisbee. Even in cycling, though your rear bears the brunt of your body weight, your feet transfer your energy to the pedals and from there to the road. If your feet are pinched, rubbing, pounded, hot, cold, slipping around, or cramping, are you going to be happy? You are not. And if you're unhappy, are you going to want to pursue your athletic dreams? Well, you may, but it's going to be harder. And since it's going to be hard enough anyway, you should remove all the obstacles you can, starting from the ground up.

Since this is a general guide to butt-kicking fitness, I'm not going to cover all the specifics of shoe buying, even for the few sports I know something about. But there are some nuggets of advice that are almost universally applicable:

Go to a store that specializes in your sport. Avoid, as much as possible, the big box sporting goods stores where the discounts are deep but the sales folk are undertrained and not overburdened with knowledge about how to fit the beginning and imperfect athlete. If you don't yet know what your sport is, look at a quality cross-training shoe that provides some cushioning for walking and moderate running and jumping, support for the side-to-side movements you would make on a court, and generally serves as an all-purpose athletic shoe. Once you find your sport, get shoes that are engineered for the demands of that sport. It really does make a huge difference.

Take the shoes for a test drive. Find a store that encourages you to try the shoes out in their natural habitat and even return them if they don't work out. If you can't go for a run or a hike in or around the retail establishment, at least simulate your chosen activity as far as possible right there in the store. And remember Chapter 1: don't worry about what anyone may think of you. Run around the display stands. Jump, squat, dance, kick, do whatever you have to do.

Order a big enough size. This is, again, primarily directed at female readers. Many women have some bizarre stigma about buying shoes in anything above a size 7. This can really come around to bite you in the ass when it comes to running shoes, which generally run at least one full size small, sometimes two. If you need a 9.5 or a 10, get it, even if you normally take an 8.5. Your toes need to breathe.

Being a girl, I could talk about shoes all day, but there are other things to consider for your overall athletic comfort. Like socks, for example. Make sure your socks are good enough to be seen with your fine shoes. No cotton tube socks. There are a lot of high-tech socks out there, and you need to find the socks that work for you. There are socks made from Smartwool (produced by sheep with exceptionally high IQs?); there are superthin, ventilating socks for cycling, double-layered blister-preventing socks, thick, cushy socks for hiking. You name it, it has probably been made into a sock. My favorite socks for both running and cycling are by DeFeet because they're thin, which gives my toes room, and they don't slip around too much in my shoes. They are also available in a variety of pleasing designs, from suns and moons to the martini glass special. But look around. Find your own socks. Remember, no cotton. Cotton gets wet, retains moisture, causes blisters. Blisters are bad.

From the bottom to the top: a few words about sports bras. Girls, take care of the girls. The only thing more discouraging than getting sore feet is having your boobs flop around like trout on a riverbank. It hurts, it makes you feel unathletic, and it makes your motion less efficient. If you are gifted in the bosom department, look at the Enell bra. Oprah loves 'em, and so do I. They aren't the cutest bras in the world, but cute is in the eye of the beholder, and boy, do these bras hold. No jiggle, no joggle. So I think they're beautiful. If you aren't so endowed that you need an Enell, at least get firm support from a reputable manufacturer. A couple more things:

First, beware of baggy shorts. If you are a person with heavy thighs (listen up, guys, this applies to you too), you are at risk of painful chafing when (not if) baggy shorts ride up on your legs. Ditch the baggies and put on the spandex. See Chapter 1 if you have objections.

Second, shop around at the discount stores and find some workout clothes made of a synthetic, wicking fabric. These go by a lot of trade names: DriFit, CoolMax, DuoFold, Thermax, and Dryline, to name a few. The idea of wicking is that the fabric's structure moves moisture away from your skin into the outer fibers of the garment. As a result, you are more comfortable and the clothing stays light rather than getting soggy and heavy with your bodily fluids. So in one fell swoop we address moisture and temperature management, as well as the ever-present threat of chafing. You may love your Def Leppard Pyromania T-shirt, but save it for that special client meeting or your first encounter with your future in-laws. Don't work out in it. All together now: "Cotton is not the workout material of choice." The reason I send you to the discount chains is that these wicking fabrics can get extra spendy, especially the ones with the fancy swoosh logos. But with a little careful shopping, you can pick up a few nice items for $10 to $20 each.

Those are the essentials. Happy feet, happy breasts, no chafing, and clothing that gets rid of your sweat. The rest of the stuff depends on your sport and your taste. One of my favorite triathlon club buddies specializes in leopard-print athletic wear. Another goes for orange everything. My favorite thing about cycling is the crazy graphics you can wear. Every Christmas, my husband, Tim, buys me an extra-cool bike jersey, like my South Park or Beatles Yellow Submarine items, and every year my mom's first words are, "Are you going to wear that?" It's all a matter of your personal style.

12

DEVELOP A MIGHTY CORE

WHILE I'VE BEEN known to rant about the idea of "body sculpting" as the center of your fitness program (see page 14), I don't want you to get the idea that you shouldn't do strength training. Far from it. Strong is good. Strong is good for men and women of all ages and shapes, and all athletic inclinations. Strong keeps you from hurting yourself; when you're hurt, you're not having fun.

And why are we hurting? Well, I'm hurting because I neglected my core. If you've been toying with the idea of committing to athletic endeavors, you may have noticed the term "core" on flyers at gyms or on fitness books. You may have heard your sporty friends bandy the word about or heard it used in connection with a Pilates class. And you may have wondered what the heck the core is.

Personal trainer, surfing coach, and author Rocky Snyder says, "The word 'core' has gotten to be overused in the health industry, and it gets muddled or confused." He explains to me that there are smaller muscles deep within the body, connected to the vertebrae, that are endurance based. These "local core" muscles have to engage before any work gets done anywhere else, and their endurance keeps you stable and balanced over the long haul. Then there are the "global core" muscles that are closer to the surface, like your abs and obliques. These muscles, says Rocky, are more dynamic and produce a lot of force compared to the local core. Most people focus on strengthening external, superficial musculature and pay less attention to the muscles deep within.

The deep muscles are the ones that will never bulge magnificently no matter how hard you "sculpt" them because they're hidden beneath other layers of muscle. Some fitness folks broaden the definition to include muscles in your hips and butt that play a huge role in stabilizing and supporting your body as it moves. I'm not qualified to make the final determination, but for me, strength and flexibility in the hip and butt regions are key to avoiding injuries.

Now, why is the core so vital? It basically holds you together, and you couldn't do much without it. Your ability to move begins at the core. If you want to raise your leg in an exuberant Rockettes kind of high kick, the brain first signals those muscles deep down under the visible muscles to contract and counterbalance the motion of all the other muscles. That way, when you deploy your leg ceilingward, you don't topple over on your heinie like some unfortunate from the Benny Hill show. The leg kick engages muscles in your abdomen, both hips, your behind, and your back. If some of those muscles are weak or tight, or if some of them are strong while others are puny, the exquisite interplay among them will break down. Then you might pull a muscle in your back, which is a painful injury, or your butt, which is an extremely embarrassing injury, or even a hip flexor, which is an extremely painful and slow-healing injury, though less embarrassing.

When the muscles of your core are strong, flexible, and developed in balance, you are fully prepared to reach your athletic potential. Your gait will be smoother; you will be more agile, more powerful, and quicker. You will be able to run longer or punch harder, or whatever it is you want to do. The joints of your legs and feet won't have to work so hard to keep you stable, so they'll be less prone to getting hurt.

Beth Rypins, an extreme world-class kayaker and raft guide, uses her core in a serious way. When she was teaching me the rudiments of paddling a kayak, she exhorted me to use the muscles of my upper back and my oblique abdominals to put power into the stroke. "Otherwise you end up 'humpin' the dog,'" she observed. This rather arcane kaykers' jargon means to try and scoot your boat forward by hunching your abdomen repeatedly in an ungainly and amusing way. Beth did not hump the dog. She was a picture of grace and power, calculation and guts as she launched herself over waterfalls and down precipitous rocky creeks. For Beth, her core was often the difference between life and death. After the birth of her daughter, however, Beth's athleticism suffered:

> I paddled hard toward the lip of the falls, leaning forward to keep my weight centered over my kayak. At the edge of the waterfall I was exactly where I wanted to be, but as I started over the edge I couldn't stay forward over my boat. Laying on the back deck instead of forward and ready to paddle, I landed at the bottom of the fifteen-foot waterfall out of control.
>
> What was wrong? Was the milk leaking from my breasts throwing off my center of gravity? Did the baby awaiting my return home distract my iron-strong attention to detail? Or did forty-one weeks of pregnancy leave my once strong six-pack in

shreds? Maybe it was a combination, but without a doubt age, pregnancy, and motherhood had softened my edge as a gnarly class V kayaker.

Pregnancy and childbirth left Beth in the common position of carrying more weight than she ever had in her life, along with the sensation of slackness in the midsection that she found disheartening. Many, many women go through this experience, but for the two-time world whitewater champion, it was particularly humbling. Now a certified personal trainer, Beth practices and teaches exercises that build from the core out and feature real-life, functional fitness rather than artificial exercises on gym machines. "In the gym, you're on a machine that works one or two muscles in isolation, not a variety of muscles all working in sync," says Beth, "whereas a functional strength workout requires you to pay attention to how different muscle groups are engaging together." Beth endorses CrossFit, an exercise approach that works every part of the body in a nonspecialized way, but the idea of building your body's core strength through exercises that use all your muscles at once is a philosophy that trumps muscle isolation. Cross Fit has its acolytes doing everything from basic gymnastics moves to sprinting to swinging "kettleball" weights around in dangerous-looking ways in order to strengthen muscles in a harmonious whole. Muscles are built to work together in complicated ways. Strengthen one group, like the big quadriceps muscles in your thighs, without strengthening the groups around them, like the hamstrings, buttocks, and hips, and you've got an injury waiting to happen.

Whatever system you pick, make sure the instructor is getting your body moving in all directions; not at once, but in some sort of sequence. Core fitness involves movements in the

THE LOWDOWN: MAKING THE WORDS REAL

So how do you go about getting yourself a mighty core, especially if you've recently given birth? First, find expert help. Don't just lie down on your living room floor and start doing endless straight-up sit-ups, because that's the kind of isolating a single muscle exercise that we want to avoid. You will develop abs at the expense of the back and sides, and your form would probably be all wrong anyway. At the very least, find a solid book on core work and develop a complete routine that works all the muscles you can't even see. But I would really recommend that you take a class. Find a gym or a fitness studio, a community college class or an offering from your local rec department. Core strength and flexibility, yoga, and Pilates all offer great approaches to making your core mighty. If you've got a bit of disposable income, find a trainer and do some one-on-one or small group work. It's well worth the investment.

Classes that develop your core musculature can include yoga, Pilates, combinations of the two, or sessions of combined strength and balance training specifically called "core fitness" or "core strengthening." Yoga has a mental/spiritual side that includes breathing deeply, sending the breath into various parts of the body, saying "ohm," and what not. Pilates (pronounced "pi-LAH-teez") is a series of highly controlled, fluid movements developed by Joseph Pilates, a self-taught movement expert who began perfecting his system while he was held in an internment camp during World War I. Core fitness or core strengthening is more sports oriented but may incorporate elements of both Pilates and yoga, along with calisthenics like push-ups and crunches.

forward and back plane, the side-to-side plane, and in rotation, like swinging a baseball bat or a golf club.

It's amazing how concentrated attention can help you learn what's going on deep in the core and identify your particular strengths and imbalances. Then you can determine the exercises that can help you get strong, stretchy, and balanced. But the key is focus and repetition, both of which you can do at home.

Here's another tip straight from the hard lessons of exercise life: if something hurts, stop doing it before it hurts more. Just because it's a core fitness class run by a qualified instructor doesn't mean you can't get injured doing it.

MOVE LIKE AN ANIMAL

SOME PEOPLE CONSIDER a ballet dancer the epitome of human grace. Others point to the gymnast as the pinnacle of the human body in motion, or to the figure skater. I feel that humans in motion should emulate animals as much as possible. Take the cat, for example. The movement of a cat is completely unstudied. When the cat darts into the house from outside, leaps up on the window sill, or just gets up from the softest spot in the house, stretches, and ambles into the kitchen to look for food, his motion is completely unselfconscious. Nothing about the cat is focused on his appearance, technique, pace, or performance. He's just going from A to B in the best way he knows how.

The only time the cat appears to be self-conscious is when he goofs—misjudges his jump to the coffee table and slides off the other side of the table in a flurry of newspapers, for example. Then he has to sit down and lick his butt furiously until you quit watching. I do not espouse this technique for avoiding self-consciousness in the human population.

But it's not just cats that look amazing in motion. A bounding Jack Russell terrier, a cutting horse working a herd of cows, a

deer on a hillside, or even a giraffe loping across the Serengeti—
all their parts move in harmony, with maximum efficiency for
their unique structure.

What makes an animal graceful? Well, lack of self-
consciousness, for one. The animal doesn't care what it looks like
in motion. This relieves the animal of unnecessary tension,
which wastes energy and is therefore inefficient. So we translate
that to human terms by focusing on relaxing every part of your
body that's not actively involved in your motion, and shedding
excess tension from body parts that are propelling you. Is focusing on relaxing a contradiction in terms? No, not at all. It's a part
of yoga, meditation, and drills that world-class athletes do to prepare themselves for a high-pressure event. You turn your attention to each part of your body and check it for tension. Then you
let the tension go. You can do this while you're moving. Un-
hunch your shoulders, shake out your arms, stretch your neck,
bring your back into an alignment that feels more balanced.

A corollary of relaxation is efficiency. Don't waste energy doing anything that doesn't move you in the direction you need to
go. Animals come by their efficiency naturally; we mostly have
to work at our motion over and over again until it feels natural.
What constitutes efficient motion varies from sport to sport.

In cycling, for example, the keys to efficiency lie in a comfortable position on the bike that allows you to generate power and a
smooth pedal stroke in which every movement of your leg con-
tributes to turning the cranks around and no movement holds the
cranks back. If this sounds puzzling, then you need to check out
some books, maybe quiz a guru at the local bike shop or even join
a bike club. You'll probably need to get the bike shop to make sure
your position on the bike is in fact comfortable and efficient. If

you dream of becoming a golfer, then efficiency is about coiling your body like a spring in your backswing and releasing that stored energy smoothly as you bring your club toward the ball.

You'll notice that I used the word "smooth" in each description of efficient motion, even though the motions are very different for cycling and golf. If your movement feels jerky while you're doing it, you're probably not being relaxed or efficient. A major reason for the breakdown of form in any sport is trying too hard. If you're running harder than you've trained yourself to run, your movement is going to look harsh and jerky. If you're overswinging on your tennis forehand or pushing too hard to get your bike up the hill, same deal. Animals rarely try too hard. I don't know if they have the mental processes that would enable them to try too hard. Their running or climbing or pouncing motions are just the ones that they've trained to do their whole lives. They're not overthinking their level of effort. And neither should you.

THE LOWDOWN: MAKING THE WORDS REAL

How exactly does one learn to move like an animal?

If you find yourself tensing up, flailing around, or losing your smoothness, just back it off a notch. Slow down.

Focus on relaxing your breathing. Identify areas of your body that are holding tension and let them relax.

Take a break. Stop and stretch. Think like a cat: any time's a good time for a stretch. Then keep going.

Picture some animal that you admire, moving in the way it moves best, and remember that the animal's not trying too hard. Picture yourself moving easily, fluidly, like the animal. You'll save yourself energy and stress, and you'll probably start feeling better and having more fun.

SWIM AT ANY OPPORTUNITY

WATER CAN SET you free from gravity in a unique way; even a heavy person can feel graceful and fluid. The water, after all, is the element of the sleek seal and the mighty whale. They have fat, sure, but they're also elegant, strong, and at ease in their element. You too can be like the mighty whale. Get into the water. You'll float. You can roll and twist and move your body in ways that are only possible in a supportive and watery environment. Even if you're not a heavy person, you can still feel the excitement and mystery of the water.

If you do carry some extra weight, you will have good buoyancy and probably good resistance to cold water as well. You will feel strong and empowered as you leap (or fall) into waters that your skinny peers eye with apprehension. If you feel nervous about water, work into it slowly. Start with the least threatening body of water you can think of, whether it's the bathtub, the kiddie pool at the YMCA, or a warm, crystal clear bit of ocean off a white sandy beach in South Maui. Whatever works.

When I was a lass, always tall for my age and always on the upper end of the "normal" weight range, I loved the water. Family legend features a hair-raising tale of me jumping into the deep end of a swimming pool at the age of two. Mom wanted Dad to jump in and rescue me, but Dad had a scientific interest in the result of my action, and sure enough, I came up dog-paddling. "Look, Ann, she's swimming," Dad said calmly. From then on it was hard to keep me out of any body of water from a puddle on up to an ocean.

Later in life, when I crept off the normal range of the weight charts and swelled inexorably toward obesity, I still took every opportunity to jump into the water. There I was unconstrained by heaviness, though sometimes by tight bathing suits. When I took up triathlon, I was delighted to have a reason to go to the pool two or three times a week, and even more delighted to have the chance to swim in open water. The water supported me; I worked on my swimming stroke to minimize its resistance and maximize my feel for the element.

"That's all very well for you," I hear you retort. "You obviously have a strong natural affinity for water. That's not true for me." Okay, I admit, it may not be true to the same degree, but I do believe that humans have affinity for water. Our bodies are largely made of water. We die from lack of water much sooner than we die from lack of food, and in fact our body and brain functions suffer quickly if the fluid balance in our body gets thrown off by 2 percent of our body weight. A couple hours of hard work in the hot sun, and you can easily be at risk for measurable cognitive impairment and physical suffering if you don't chug your aqua with proper electrolyte supplementation, as described in Chapter 20. So we're very dependent on our internal water. We also come from a watery prenatal environment, enveloped in a snug sac of fluids, getting our oxygen not from air but directly from mom's blood. Without getting all New Age, I feel that I can safely say that we have strong innate ties to water and that exploring the nature of those ties can teach us interesting things about ourselves.

When you start exploring different kinds of aquatic environments, you learn what you're afraid of. And that's always useful. Some people are afraid of slimy things; others don't like the idea of things with teeth. Other folks are nervous about water they can't see the bottom of. Some people fear open water in an unspecified way. There are granite-rimmed alpine lakes up at around 10,000 feet, but some people are afraid of freezing their goolies off in high mountain water. There's also salt, chlorine, and the fear of simply plummeting to the bottom of whatever water it is.

It's not surprising that water is as scary as it is attractive, as overwhelming as it is liberating. Water can be impenetrable, implacable, destructive, enormously powerful, tossing huge objects around like toys. It is the surge of a giant hurricane, the churn of the rapid, the towering wave that dwarfs the fragile ship. Every swimmer knows these images, this power, and we all should. Swimming without respect for the water is a mug's game.

We do a lot of things that involve forces more powerful than ourselves. We drive around in hurtling metal monsters, fly in steel tubes six miles up in the air, operate gas stoves, expose our tender brains to television. So I invite you to do the same thing with the water. Be smart and alert, as you are when you're driving or cooking. Then trust that the water will hold you, and that the creatures living in it have no particular interest in doing anything but staying out of your way. Fall into the great rocking cradle of the world. Kick your legs, move your arms around. Breathe. Go swimming.

THE LOWDOWN: MAKING THE WORDS REAL

Are you one of those people who start to hyperventilate at the idea of putting your head in the water? If you are truly phobic, you probably need professional help to work at desensitizing yourself to the fear. If you're more nervous than paralyzed by fear, though, here are some ideas for acclimating yourself to the life aquatic.

Get a water buddy. Find someone who will support and encourage you but not push you too far beyond your comfort zone. This should probably be someone who knows what it's like to feel nervous about water, not a seal in human clothing who'll be all, "Come *on!* It's just water! It's nothing to be afraid of!"

Get your feet wet. Then your knees. Hang out with your water buddy while you sit on the steps of the pool (or on the lake shore, or whatever body of water represents the scary kind of water). Then graduate to standing and walking around in the water. Breathe deeply. Visualize things that make you feel safe and strong.

Put your face in the water. A scuba mask can help with this, making your face and eyes feel less vulnerable. Do this until it no longer seems scary. Take as much time as you need. Weeks, months, whatever.

Learn to float. Have your water buddy support your back while you lean backward into the water and raise your feet off the bottom. Breathe deeply and feel how the air in your lungs makes you float higher in the water.

If you know how to swim but lake water freaks you out, try going through these steps in a lake as though you were learning to swim for the first time. If you don't know how to swim, go through these steps until you feel comfortable with them. Then learn to dog-paddle with your water buddy. Next you can get into a class and learn a couple of strokes. Finally, you can get out of the parking lot and onto the open road, or, in this case, into the open water. Don't swim alone, follow the surf advisories and stay out of rapids unless you have a life jacket and some safety kayakers to pick you up at the bottom.

15

EMBRACE YOUR BODILY FLUIDS

ALL ATHLETES SWEAT, even the perfect ones. In fact, the perfect ones sweat copious amounts when they are doing their athletic thing. Sweating is how your body maintains its temperature in a healthy range, and it is also a vital part of the complex system of eliminating waste materials from the body. I admired a recent series of Gatorade ads showing athletes sweating prodigiously, with brightly colored Gatorade emanating from their pores. The ads featured seriously sweating women athletes alongside the men. Those women were sweating big time, and it looked great. Back in the bad old days, societal norms forbade women to appear to sweat, even when playing tennis, which was about the only athletic activity that grown women were encouraged to do, as far as I can tell. Betty Crocker did not sweat, ever, no matter how much she baked. Women simply did not sweat until about 1982.

I have always sweated. At school recess and lunch, I would get so hot and sweaty playing basketball or handball that my glasses would remain fogged up the rest of the day (it's surprising I learned anything). I never worried too much about my tendency toward abundant glowing. I was way too busy worrying, when I became old enough to worry about my appearance, about boobs, zits, braces, and overall body shape. Besides, I was good at sports that didn't involve running too fast or too far, so sweating during strenuous sporting activity became equivalent with fun. And while many of my core tenets have changed since I was twelve (thankfully), I'm still perfectly at ease with sweating while exercising.

But a lot of women, I notice, still don't think it's good to sweat. It's unfeminine, they think. You don't look good sweating, they think. It makes your makeup run and reduces your 'do to a bedraggled mop. I have had women tell me that they "hate to sweat." Well, what did we talk about in Chapter 8? Not hating. If you "hate to sweat," you hate how you feel when you sweat. Now that can be a purely physical thing—you feel slimy, drippy, squishy, or unpleasant in some other way. If your dislike of sweating stems from physical discomfort, there are some apparel adjustments that may help. Dress lightly, even if you feel exposed. Better to show your thunder thighs to the whole planet than to suffer in heavy sweatpants; that's what the *Slow Fat Triathlete* counsels. Wear wicking fabrics that help your sweat get off of your skin so the clothes dry faster. Make sure that you maintain vigilance against glow-induced chafing: unguents such as Aquaphor, BodyGlide, or plain old Vaseline applied to your hot spots will help immeasurably. (See Chapter 22 for more on hot spots and how to soothe them.) Keep a towel handy and wear a headband if sweat runs into your eyes. Drink ample amounts of fluids, so that the fluid out is more or less replaced by fluid in. Getting the water/sports drink into your gullet will help you avoid the fatigue and discomfort that come with dehydration.

If you do all this and you still feel uncomfortable sweating, I have only one piece of advice: suck it up, cupcake. You want to be an athlete, and athletes sweat. Learn to love sweating. Embrace your sweat; revel in it. See it as tangible evidence of your effort and your burgeoning athleticism. As you become a more advanced sweater, um, person who sweats, you may even wish to attempt to spit unobtrusively during selected outdoor workouts. It's icky, but sometimes you really need to.

Same advice goes out to all you other cupcakes (and I use the term with complete affection) who feel anxious or embarrassed by sweating. Get over it. Please. Refer yet again to Chapter 1 and my sermonizing on self-consciousness and the evils thereof. You have a right to sweat. Of course, you owe it to society and to yourself to maintain high standards of hygiene before and after your workout, and if you do so, even during your workout you will be reasonably acceptable in terms of stinkiness. You'll just be wet, and a bit salty. That's not gross or disgusting, and it doesn't make you a Bad Person. It may, however, make you an athlete.

16

BE INCONSISTENT

OOPS. I MEANT to say "Be consistent." Didn't I? Isn't consistency the hallmark of champions? And even of ordinary shlubs like us who pursue great athletic goals? Don't you need to dedicate yourself to your athletic dreams, day in, day out, week after week, month after month, year after year? Well, yes. But also no. Yes, you should be doing something active four to six days a week. But *not* seven. Seven is right out. You need a rest day. Even God needed a rest day.

But a slavish dedication to consistency may turn into boredom, especially if you specialize in one activity like running. For example: Monday, rest. Tuesday, speed run. Wednesday, easy run. Thursday, medium distance run. Friday, rest. Saturday, run long and easy. Sunday, run easy and short. I actually like running, even though I suck at it, and I engaged in a regimen somewhat like that for five months or so while marathon training. But there is a certain monotony inherent in the system. Plod, plod, plod along the streets, sidewalks, trails, and multiuse paved paths of Mountain View and its environs. Plod, plod, plod. I sought out different routes and practiced being in the moment in a very Zen way, but frankly, I was ready to mix in other sports by the time I recovered from the marathon. Even if you're training for a marathon, there's no reason you can't mix in a swim, a bike ride, or a vigorous session of catch. Sometimes—and guru of the balanced workout Rocky Snyder would argue often—your body and your mind will benefit more from mixing in a different activity and not doing the scheduled run.

Some people thrive on routine. I am not one of them, and you may not be either. A lot of people who write about fitness recommend working different activities into your repertoire. There are several reasons for this. First, you work and rest different muscles, joints, and tendons when you change activities, making you a more balanced athlete and less prone to overuse injuries. Second, your brain stays fresh. Third, you can buy more clothes. (I know, I said earlier that it's not about the gear, but I totally lied. I love buying sports gear. Love it, love it, love it.)

Rocky Snyder, the aforementioned author, surfer, snowboarder, kayaker, and personal trainer who specializes in being unspecialized, is a huge advocate of moving around in different ways. He recommends adding exercises and sports that involve lateral and rotational movement, like tennis, skating, African or hip-hop dance, basketball—anything to get out of that straight line rut. "Runners," says Rocky, "are the worst. They're like heroin addicts. If they're running, they're happy, but you can't get them to do anything but run." If you want to focus on becoming a better runner, you would do well to run less and do a couple of cross-training workouts on those days you're not running. You might get faster. You might easily stay uninjured for longer, and injuries are always lurking in the shadows, waiting to pounce on athletes who do lots and lots of one thing and not enough other things to balance that one thing. You know what I mean. If you're not focused on being a better runner or a better cyclist, or a better single-sport specialist, then it's that much easier to be unspecialized.

The threat of workout boredom can strike the beginning athlete or the seasoned veteran alike. Two-time world whitewater champion Beth Rypins trained her butt off for years to stay in top shape for her extreme adventures. Eventually age and the demands of motherhood ate into her commitment. "My body won't hold up, I'm tired of it, it's boring," she informed me with typical candor. Her solution was to specialize in unspecialized fitness through CrossFit's short yet intense workout of jumping, sprinting, weights, and other varieties of fun.

You don't have to be super intense, though. You can kick ass by mixing things up. Nadya in Albany has plans to put together a women's fitness group that tries a different sport every Saturday: basketball, tai chi, volleyball, rowing, badminton—whatever the members decide. She plans to call it SNARL: Subversive Neo-Athletes Reclaiming Lycra. You could develop your own SNARL franchise, or you could do your own individual snarl. Become a swimmer for three months: immerse yourself in swimming (so to speak). Then metamorphose into a ballroom dancer for four months. Then give aikido your all.

My one caveat to this approach is that you should make your first sports rotation a good four-month sequence in core strength and flexibility (for a refresher course on the importance of core, go back to Chapter 12), maybe something like CrossFit. The really short version is this: a good core program strengthens all the muscle groups that hold your body in good alignment when you move, improves your balance, increases your power, and (always key for any athlete, especially the imperfect ones) reduces risk of injury. Core: good. Injury: bad. Core work and mixing up your activities complement each other perfectly.

Or you can be inconsistent in a more impromptu way, even within your routine. Some examples:

You could go to the gym intending to do twenty minutes on the treadmill and a circuit of strength training, but then experience a sudden urge to mix it up with jazz aerobics. Let me first warn you that if you walk all unprepared into a jazz aerobics class, you may end up crossing your feet and falling down in front of a whole group of lithe dancer types, but that's not so bad.

Try a different weight machine, possibly the one with the weird wings sticking out on the side that you could never figure out what it was for. Ask someone to show you.

Ask the gym staff to show you some exercises with free weights. A lot of us imperfect female athletes shy away from free weights because we weren't taught to work with them in school and they seem scary and testosterone laden. But they are more helpful than weight machines for developing real-world strength and balance.

And speaking of balance, there's nothing as goofy and as useful as those giant rubber balance balls. They can help you develop strong, stable muscles in all the important areas of your abdomen, back, hips, and butt. Even work that hurts your tummy muscles is less onerous when a giant rubber ball is involved. If you don't know how to make the most of them, ask your helpful gym staff.

Go out for a bike ride on a sunny day and ditch the gym altogether.

You don't have to have an overarching athletic goal to be an athlete. It doesn't make you any more imperfect if you choose not to specialize at all. In fact, according to the folks at CrossFit and other cross-training fitness programs, being a little good at a variety of disciplines can make you very, very fit overall. For me, having a big hairy anxiety-producing athletic goal like a marathon or riding the classic climbs of the Tour de France is a fun thing, but it's not the only way to go. Or you could set a big hairy goal that involves engaging in twelve different activities in a calendar year. The only consistency that matters is that you have a good time moving your butt on a regular basis.

THE LOWDOWN: MAKING THE WORDS REAL

Here's a sample schedule for someone who wants to build a multifaceted structure of inconsistency, with the goal of being more active and having more fun. Notice how we're balancing aerobic activity (swimming, jogging, cycling, hiking) with core strength and flexibility (Yoga, Pilates, or strength training); solitary activities with family outings and group activities; structured classes or workouts with freewheeling fun. Notice too how we're not following core strength activities with more core strength, or endurance with more endurance. Also notice that this isn't really about getting you up the hill, mountain, or mound of your choice, just about moving.

Monday	Tuesday	Wednesday	Thursday	Friday	Saturday
Week 1					
Rest. Starting work week is hard enough.	Relaxed 30-min. swim.	Yoga/Pilates or other core fitness class.	Slightly less relaxed 30-min. swim.	Walk, jog, or bike for 20–30 min. Follow with 30 min. of yoga or other core on your own.	Bike or hike with the family (or without them)—as many minutes as you like.
Week 2					
Rest. Maybe stretch a bit if you feel stiff.	Jog or bike 20–30 min., followed by strength training.	Swim as far as you want.	Yoga/Pilates or core fitness.	Go out dancing. It's Friday! Or take an aerobics class.	Sleep late. Play a game later if you feel like it.
Week 3					
More resting. Mmm.	Yoga/Pilates or core.	Walk, jog, bike for 30–40 min.	Yoga/Pilates or core.	Swim, bike, or jog. Or nap.	Spend the day at the park. Play as many games as you can.
Week 4					
Yoga/Pilates or core.	Take a nap or stretch.	20–30 min. cardio (bike, jog, walk), then 30–40 min. core/strength.	Dance class.	Take the day off. (Take an extra rest every 4–5 weeks.)	Hike or bike, with or without people.

17

GO OUTSIDE

I AM LUCKY enough to live in an extremely moderate climate. It rains in the winter, and the weather is sometimes chilly and windy. Occasionally, during a cold snap, puddles freeze overnight, and you have to watch your step. In the summer, the natural air conditioning of the Pacific Ocean keeps the temperatures from getting too high, and we have low humidity. Life is good and comfortable here in Mountain View. And yet people persist on exercising indoors here in weather that Midwesterners would consider a Must Go Outside sort of a day. Now, the gym holds an important place in the imperfect athlete's fitness repertoire. Sometimes, and especially in some places, it's way too nasty to be outside. It's too cold, too dark, too sketchy in the neighborhood, or too iced-over with the remnants of last night's ice storm. Also, the gym usually has a lot better weight equipment than you do at home, and sometimes even a pool. Oh, and the Jacuzzi, which is actually my favorite thing about the gym. Plus the gym has child care, which is helpful if you have a child or two. Maybe you have a perfect gym routine down. You always go when there's no wait for the machines; you have a slammin' mix of tunes on your iPod. You get on that treadmill and you get into a zone, in a world of your own, feeling no pain. It's excellent if it works, and you look forward to that zone every time you go; it is absolutely awesome.

When the gym routine starts feeling stale, however, try going outside. Explore. Outside has air and trees, and houses with gardens or fun blocks full of interesting stores or gently curving streets with parks or whatever. Outside has variety and things to look at and smells that change with the seasons and the piles of garbage in the back alleys (ooh, bad example). Outside is a less controlled environment. It forces you to adapt to the unexpected, like small variations in terrain, like the weather, like seed pods under your wheels.

It's not just my personal preference for outside versus inside that lies beneath this hypothesis. There's like, psychology and stuff that we can talk about. I have an awesome book called *The Non-Runner's Marathon Trainer*, based on this incredibly successful class at the University of Northern Iowa called Marathon 101. Students and members of the public entered a lottery to get into the sixteen-week class, which was essentially training for a marathon. The professors, one from the physical education department and one from psychology, put together a combination of mental and physical preparation that enabled 199 out of 200 first-time marathon runners to finish the marathon at the end of the class. (The 200th person got dehydrated; see Chapter 20.)

I used the training schedule as a guideline and mixed it up with a couple other training plans, but what I really enjoyed was the mental part of the preparation. One chapter talks about associative and dissociative techniques for coping with training for a staggeringly long event. Dissociate is what you do if you put yourself in the controlled environment of the gym and use some means of disconnecting your mind from what your body is doing. Listening to music, reading magazines, watching TV if you have a swankified health club and not a gym, or even just drifting off into lottery winner fantasies. Nothing wrong with this.

Associative techniques, on the other hand, are what bring you into intense, focused concentration on what your body is doing, and what your mind is doing while your body is working. Chapter 50 focuses on mental techniques and training your brain to appreciate what your body's up to. But let's just focus for now on what being outside does in that regard. If you're running outside, you have to focus in order to avoid uneven pavement and other obstacles, to step on and off the curbs, to dodge slower or faster pedestrians and baby joggers. You become aware that you're on a slight uphill grade or a slight downhill; that you're running into the wind or with the wind at your back. You're in the real world, with your real body, and you are forced to pay attention to both.

And—forgive me, treadmill devotees—it's just way less boring to be outside.

I know from my experiences as a traveling Russian-language interpreter (a past life) and from my imperfectly athletic friends around the country that outdoor exercise can in fact take place in pretty extreme conditions. Okay, maybe you can't play tennis when there's three feet of snow on the ground, but you can snowshoe, right? The mental toughness and confidence you gain from pulling on a couple of layers of workout clothes, a neck gaiter, hat and gloves and heading out into a seemingly inhospitable environment will serve you extremely well down the road when you come up against some challenging conditions in a race or other workout. Knowing you went out when the mercury stood at 20 degrees can give you a serious edge when you head out for your 10k in May and it's raining.

Even if your sports of choice are primarily indoor-oriented, I invite you to put your nose outside the door once in a while.

THE LOWDOWN: MAKING THE WORDS REAL

Here are some suggestions for the occasional outdoor excursion:

Coach extraordinaire Lisa Engles suggests, "Look at the outside world as your gym. Look at a tree stump as a place to do step ups. See a stair railing as a place to do a set of push-ups or stretches. It makes it like a treasure hunt."

In fact, do a treasure hunt. Make up a series of clues for your friends to figure out in the swanky suburb, or downtown early on a Sunday morning. Ask them what animal adorns the gateposts at 284 Elm Street, or the name of the building at 222 South 22nd Street. Divvy the friends up into teams. First team in with all the clues wins a prize. Requires some homework, but really, really good times can be had.

Drive to a swanky suburban neighborhood on a weekend morning. Do your walking or running there. Find a hillier or flatter neighborhood than you're used to.

The more obvious options: go to a park, a beach, a hill, a lakeside path, the dog park. Even if you don't have a dog, you can run around and the doggies can chase you, which is really fun for them. You don't have to do this stuff every day, just once in a while. Make a treat out of it. Take a picnic for when you're tired of moving. Bring the whole family.

Take off your stinky hand wraps and boxing gloves and go for a walk or a bike ride, or go play volleyball in the park with your friends. Put down your squash racquet and go rent a sea kayak or a canoe with your husband or your girlfriend. Remember, inconsistency is good for us. It keeps us fresh and motivated, and it uses our minds and bodies in new ways.

Go outside. Even if you hate it, at least you'll appreciate your cozy treadmill all the more once you get back in the gym. But you might not hate it. You might have a little fun. Being indoors is what enabled the development of civilization, but being outside is what makes humans athletes.

TAKE TWO STEPS BACK, ONE STEP FORWARD

I SEE THE skeptical eyebrow you are raising at me. This does not sound like a tip for ass-kicking fitness, you are thinking. This sounds like a recipe for a sense of frustration and failure. Which it is. But true ass-kicking fitness embraces frustration and failure, which are as inevitable as the Cubs failing to win the World Series. And after you accept these negative and unpleasant feelings, you can go ahead and take your next step forward.

At some point, your transformation into a joyful, shame-free, butt-kicking athlete will be rudely interrupted. You will pull a muscle badly and go "Ow. Ow. Ow ow ow!" Or you will strain your back, catch the flu, get sent out of town on business for a month, or have to drive your kids to soccer so often that all you can do is work, drive, and sleep. Your progress will stall. You will get frustrated. You may even miss the schedule for some of your intermediate goals, like the momentous day when you jog two miles, or even a big goal, like your first tae kwon do bout. You may go back to the couch for a time and wallow in a slough of despond, which translates into watching endless reruns of *Law and Order*. Or *South Park*, or *Frasier*. That's okay. It's normal.

In the seven years or so since I started on the road to permanent athleticism, I have strained my back twice and my neck at least once; suffered a hip flexor injury that took six months to heal completely and still bothers me from time to time; gotten at least three nasty bouts of bronchitis and two of food poisoning; had an inflammation of the Achilles tendon; acquired a painful right shoulder (not the same shoulder I had operated on in 1997); and experienced a relapse of repetitive strain injury in my wrists. Nothing terrible, nothing overly traumatic, but stuff that put me on that couch, sometimes for a couple of weeks at a time. And I would wallow, and I would indulge in my own set of wallowing-related vices, which tend to include overproduction and subsequent overconsumption of buttered toast in addition to the compulsive viewing of police procedurals.

However, the reason that I am still an ass-kicking athlete is that I would get back up and take another step forward. Even if it meant starting again almost from square one. When my hip flexor was hurting so badly that I couldn't run and could hardly walk for exercise, I got in the pool. When I couldn't actually kick my legs either, I got a leg buoy (this is a cute little floaty foam hourglass-shaped thing that you clamp between your thighs in a very attractive way) and swam like that. When I got a sore shoulder, I swam backstroke, which didn't hurt, until it didn't hurt to swim frontstroke anymore. Yeah, I know "frontstroke" isn't a word, but I think it should be. Anyhow, it's way better than "breaststroke," wouldn't you agree?

When you're hurt or sick or frazzled from work or family crap, you have to get creative, and you have to get very determined. You have to hang on to your vision of yourself as an athlete, of someone who is worthy of being an athlete and cannot be stopped from doing the things that athletes do. You have to be a pit bull on your own pant leg. Grab onto that inner athlete and do not let go no matter what happens. Sneak in a session of late night headphone disco dancing, just you and your iPod, if you haven't had time to work out in two weeks. Put a fake meeting on your Outlook and go to the pool instead. (Don't forget the hair dryer.) Walk if you can't run; do crunches if you can't walk; stretch the parts it doesn't hurt to stretch; ride the stationary bike easy for twenty minutes instead of going for two hours up Nasty-Ass Hill. Do something. Anything.

You have to strike a delicate balance between being determined and being patient if your body is hurt or sick. Keep a leash on that pit bull so you don't end up hurting yourself or getting sicker. Rule of thumb if you're sick: don't exercise if you have a fever, sore throat, or chest congestion, or if you feel too lousy to get out of bed. You're sick for a reason. Rest until you feel a bit of energy coming back. Rule of thumb if you're hurt: push a little. Just a little. If you have sharp pain in a joint or tendon, stop. If you feel sore or stiff, go easy. Put an ice pack on the sore part when you're done (15 to 20 minutes, no more) and take your over-the-counter anti-inflammatory drug of choice. If it hurts worse after two days, you overdid it. Recalibrate, rest, and try again when the hurt calms down. If it hurts again, see your doctor.

Healing is part of becoming an athlete. Every time you work out, you are injuring yourself very slightly. You are stressing muscle fibers and connective tissue. You're even causing little tears in your muscles. When you rest enough between workouts, those tears and strains heal and the muscles and tendons become stronger and more resilient. When you don't rest enough, you get hurt. So judicious use of rest in order to heal is a critical part, maybe the most critical part, of learning to use your body effectively. It's hard to be patient when the healing has to take a while. I get crabby and sluggish and sometimes I despair of ever feeling fit and fluid again. But that feeling does come back. Maybe your first easy workout after the setback will feel like dooky. Maybe the second one too. But eventually you will feel it again: that exhilarating sense that your body is moving as nature intended.

The Breathless Mermaids are a small, informal triathlon training group formed by three women in their thirties and forties. Mary Jane Zanelli, teacher, community activist, and history buff, almost became a little too breathless during her quest to finish her first triathlon:

About a year ago my friend Nadya asked if I was interested in doing a triathlon. Between hitting middle age, heading toward menopause, becoming too busy to move, and taking on more of my fun-loving Tyrolean grandmother's physique, I thought it was a crazy idea, but then . . .

Along my sojourn back to moving I encountered some doubting people, others who said 'yeah right' with just a look, but more often people who were excited. On this quest for moving freely, I took to heart the advice of listening to your body, especially after a month of training when I did not feel quite right. My doctor told me my blood pressure was a little high and to stop all activity. I did and then for some reason, after monitoring the blood pressure for a month, it was normal again. I went on my merry way to continue training.

That March my partner Susan and I went to Virgin Gorda. About twenty minutes into a daylong snorkel trip, I started to feel a bit off. I thought maybe I was getting seasick because the water was moving me around. Again, I listened to my body, and it was saying get out of the water NOW! By the time I reached the boat, I was shaking and felt light-headed. My breathing was irregular, and I was paler than a flounder. The captain had me rushed to the clinic on the island. The doctor gave some meds to get my blood pressure down. Once again I had to stop training for over a month. No one knows why my blood pressure was acting up, but it got itself back on track. Some people thought I might not be able to compete in the triathlon after missing another month of training. What they forgot is that I was not competing, I was participating. I was not in this to set a record or to place (I came in last, as it happened). I was there to move, be part of something, relive memories of being a kid again when we swam, biked, and ran around all day, every day. One of the worst things I could do was not to try. So I "tri-ed" not once but twice, and I will keep on "tri-ing" because it is fun!

Have faith: in most cases, sickness, injury, and insane life situations are temporary. You can battle back. Just keep moving and never give up on yourself. Ever.

TAP INTO SOME AGGRO

I'**M NOT ADVOCATING** anything that would get you arrested. I'm thinking of tapping into the power of aggression from an athletic standpoint. I think that aggression and physical contact, properly managed, can be great fun and very useful to emerging athletes. The surge of energy you get when you're involved in an actual physical struggle with another person can teach you lots of new things about yourself. When you learn to tap into how much you want to run through that line, land that uppercut, make that tackle, get that rebound—embrace that "urrgggghhh!" surge of aggression—you can do more, go farther, work harder.

As a college senior, I was a charter member of the Radcliffe Rugby Club. We didn't have many practices before our first real match, a road trip out to Holy Cross in the charming burg of Worcester, Massachusetts. But that was okay because it wasn't much of a match. We lined up for the kickoff on what appeared to be a cow pasture, but I was pumped. I was about to become a rugby player. Roo, who played flanker beside me in the scrum, suffered from some trepidation. "We're going to get our bones crushed!" she warbled in a mock-tremulous falsetto. "Bones crushed!" I tried to assure her that it was we who would be crushing bones. Toward the end of the match, with no bones yet crushed, the ball bounced into my hands around the Holy Cross twenty-meter line. There were no speedy backs for me to toss the ball to, so I started to rumble forward on my own, gaining a few yards before the opponents caught up with me.

One woman grabbed me and tried to pull me down, then another, but I kept staggering forward. My teammates ran up behind me and "bound on," locking their arms around me and pushing the opposing tacklers. I held onto the ball as if it was made of gold and howled, "Push! PUSH!" We kept moving forward, pushing them back toward their own try line. I was surrounded by a heaving mass of sweaty women, half of them clawing at the ball, the other half pushing at my back. I was straining, grunting, pushing, leaning, and then I could see the try line. I lunged, quivering with effort, forcing the whole mass of womanity across the line. I fell to the ground with the ball clutched to my chest. Approximately fourteen young women, some of them built like me, fell on top of me. The ball contacted my solar plexus with a nauseating impact, and I lay paralyzed, unable to take a breath, filled with an overpowering sense of triumph. I had scored a try, and the match was over. It was ugly, ungraceful, and yes, it was violent. But man, it was fun. And that struggle, the aggression of combat, proved to be a seminal moment for me, a memory I use as a symbol for really, really wanting something, wanting it badly enough to push other people around for it. They had agreed to the pushing around by being on the pitch, and they were pushing me around too, so the violence was all fair play.

Why is embracing violence or aggression a good thing for an athlete? Obviously if you're a boxer or martial artist, you have to be willing to hit, grab, or throw someone, and the more willing you are to do that, the better you can be. In rugby, basketball, or even soccer, if you're not ready to bang bodies with the other gals or guys, you're not going to be playing the game to its fullest. Sport evolved out of prehistoric competitions that kept us sharp for the serious business of tracking, hunting, and, yes, killing other beings. Sports and violence are inextricably linked down at their murky, primal sources.

Modern Americans are rarely required to hunt for food or defend ourselves or our tribe. The closest we get to outright aggression is pounding on the steering wheel when some idiot cuts us off. In traffic, aggression does not serve us well; a Zen approach is far more effective at preserving our safety and our sanity. But aggression does serve us in our sporting endeavors.

If your sports of choice don't involve contact or even head-to-head competition, you can still channel aggression to bust out of your self-imposed limitations. A hill can be the enemy. Grit your teeth, narrow your eyes into a steely gaze, and attack. Stomp on that hill. Make it submit to your will. Show it who's boss. Take out all the anger that you can muster and pedal or run up that thing like it was trying to steal your lunch. The power of your rage, your urge to conquer and annihilate, your inner violence can get you up that hill faster than you ever believed possible.

Violence can be your friend—in sports. How do you tap into your inner aggression and use it to become a better athlete? First, find what makes you mad. For me it tends to be traffic and work-related issues. If you have spent your entire life tamping down your anger and not expressing it, this part could be a little scary. Come at it sideways. Think, "If I were queen of the universe, I would punish _____ for doing _____ ." I bet you can find something that gets you frothing at the mouth, metaphorically speaking. Next, go do your exercise of choice or try a new one. If you're youngish and resilient, try rugby or boxing or kickboxing for a change of pace. If you're oldish and less resilient, just try some pounding on the heavy bag with hand wraps and proper gloves. Go to a batting cage or driving range and hit fifty balls as hard as you can. Even if you miss the balls entirely, swinging that bat or club with a monumental grunt will be a good start.

Remember the things that make you mad and put all your energy into annihilating them through your sport. If you've got a bat or a club in your hand, pretend you're swinging at your computer monitor or your fifteen-year-old's stereo. That should tap into your internal rage. If you're on a bike, put that aggressive energy into some surges of fast pedaling. If you're lifting weights, finish off each rep with a snarl. It can be a silent snarl if you're embarrassed about snarling in public.

Please note that I'm not advocating playing your sport in a constant frenzy of anger. It's not enjoyable, and it can interfere with other things you need to be effective, like smoothness, relaxation, and awareness of the moment. Practice aggression occasionally so you can find ways to tap into the aggression when you need it: for that steep hill, that key rebound, that last lunge.

SECTION III

EIGHT WAYS TO CARE FOR YOUR BODY

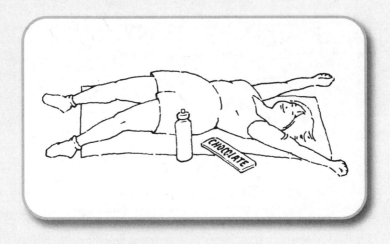

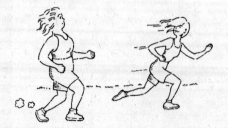

HYDRATE, HYDRATE, HYDRATE (BUT NOT TOO MUCH)

TIM, WHO HAS a healthy skepticism when it comes to received wisdom or assumptions of all kinds, believes that Americans are overly obsessed with drinking water. He says he can't find the origin of the oft repeated health advice that everyone should drink eight glasses of water each day, at least. So my friends and I—all firm believers in the general benefits of lots of cool, clean water—got onto the trusty Internet to find the science behind the adage that the average adult needs eight cups of water daily. To our surprise, we found articles saying, "Nobody knows for sure where the 8 x 8 ounces of water dictum comes from." One *Los Angeles Times* article quoted a nutrition researcher as saying, "I can't even tell you that, and I've written a book on water."

Some hypotheses are that the measurements come from the average fluid intake and output of hospital patients, or from studies showing that the average adult produces 1.5 liters of urine a day. (Really? Man, that seems like a whole lotta pee to me.) Plus, of course, what you lose through sweat and bowel movements. But the 8 x 8 rule is a general rule of thumb, and it's definitely not an absolute minimum. The same *L.A. Times* article quoted a kidney specialist at the National Institutes for Health as saying that an average-size healthy adult with healthy kidneys sitting in a temperate climate needs no more than one liter of fluid to replace what is lost during the day. So that's like four cups, plus a bit extra for that silly metric system. And unless you live on potato chips and beef jerky, you probably replace a certain amount of that fluid through the food you eat.

Until recently I took as an article of faith that caffeinated beverages don't count toward fluid replacement because they have a diuretic effect. Tim and I argued about this for years, actually. He said, look, the cup of coffee is eight ounces of water with some coffee flavors and caffeine in it. Are you telling me that you will be more dehydrated if you drink eight ounces of coffee than if you drank no fluid at all? Will the coffee actually cause you to pee out nine ounces of urine? Uh, yeah, something like that, I would say, even though it didn't quite make sense to me.

During the great hydration research project, we found studies indicating that caffeinated beverages have little to no dehydrating effect, particularly on people who are used to consuming them. So then I quit obsessing about whether I was getting my 8 x 8, and whether my cup of black tea in the morning canceled out one of my glasses of water. I still like drinking water and probably average between four and eight cups on an average sedentary day. And I am learning, slowly, to check facts carefully before debating my husband.

But there are a couple of key qualifiers about the amount of fluid adults need. An "average-size" adult, "sitting" (not exercising) in a "temperate climate." Exercise increases your need to consume fluids. When you exercise, you sweat. The more you exercise, the more you sweat. Some people sweat more than others and need to drink more to replace those fluids. Serious athlete geeks, especially those who engage in lengthy bouts of exercise, say two or three hours' worth, often weigh themselves before and after exercise (buck nekkid, so as to negate the weight of water retained in workout clothes), tallying up the fluid consumed during exercise and calculating the net fluid loss during the exercise session. So say you weighed 165 before your two-hour bike ride and 164 after. That's 16 ounces lost. But you also consumed 24 ounces of fluid during the ride, so you really lost 40 ounces of fluid total, or 20 ounces per hour. Theoretically, if you made sure to drink 20 ounces for each hour you rode, you would show no change on the scale after your ride. Of course, that would vary some from ride to ride, depending on the weather, your effort level, your salt intake, and a bunch of other factors.

I have never reached this lofty level of geekiness; I just try and drink plenty of fluids before, during, and after exercise. I also make sure that my fluids contain electrolytes. If you sweat out sodium and potassium, and trust me, you do, those minerals need to be replaced or you can really mess yourself up. I'm not talking here about a twenty-minute walk around the block, or even a forty-minute jaunt around the neighborhood on your beach cruiser bike. I'm talking more about moderate to intense effort lasting well over an hour. There have been some heavily publicized warnings recently about the dangers of hyponatremia, otherwise known as "water intoxication," which apparently affects folks like marathon runners and triathletes more severely and frequently than dehydration does. If you sweat out electrolytes and take in just water, you're not replacing the electrolytes, which are crucial to the regulation of your nervous system. Your brain and your heart depend on those electrolytes being in balance. The sodium situation is particularly dire.

So if you're going out to sweat for two or three hours, get yourself some electrolyte replacement. This comes in many forms, from the readily available Gatorade to the more specialized Cytomax or Accelerade or any number of drinks and powders you can buy at the sports store. See the sidebar on the next page for more details.

My rule of thumb is that I should return from my bout of exercise and pee copiously right away. If I'm having to stop every half hour to pee while exercising, I'm probably drinking too much. If I come back from a vigorous three-hour bike ride and I don't have to pee for two hours afterward, I'm not drinking enough. I also check out the color of the pee. Light yellow = good. Dark yellow = bad. I once read a book claiming that the well-hydrated athlete's urine should be "straw colored." I'm thinking, what, I should keep a basket of freshly cut oat straw next to my toilet like a color swatch?

In the end, it doesn't have to be rocket science. Drink when you're thirsty. Drink more when you sweat more. If you sweat a lot for a long time, get electrolytes into your bod.

THE LOWDOWN: MAKING THE WORDS REAL

Despite my newfound skepticism about the need to drink, drink, drink, I do try and consume plenty of fluids and electrolytes, especially if I'm out for a long time in the heat. Gatorade is the best-known electrolyte replacement, and if you tolerate it during long, hard exercise, stick with it. If it messes with your digestion, though, try some other options. Sports stores carry a selection of powdered mixes like Cytomax, Accelerade, GU$_2$O Hydration Drink, Amino Vital, PowerBar Endurance, and so on. Try them in sample sizes until you find one you like that sits well in your stomach while you're moving vigorously.

You can also buy electrolyte tablets that are taken with plain water or dissolved in water. Some people even drink Pedialyte, the stuff you give your little kids when they have diarrhea. I like Cytomax myself, but the key is to find something you like and drink plenty of it.

FUEL YOURSELF, SUGAR

SUGAR IS WHAT it's all about. And I'm not speaking here merely as a lifelong donut junkie. Sugar is what drives every single thing your body does, from the flight of your fingers over the keyboard to the superhuman effort of sprinting up a steep hill to calling up the memory of your first kiss. None of it could happen without sugar. And a certain amount of fat too. The fuel that activates your muscles is, under most circumstances, a combination of sugar and fat.

To be more exact, I'm not talking about C & H pure cane table sugar. Nor am I talking about brown sugar (regular sugar with molasses), powdered sugar, corn syrup, or beet sugar.

There are lots of kinds of sugar. I'm talking about glucose, which is the form of sugar that your body produces when it breaks down the diverse stuff you eat: porterhouse steaks, Cheez Whiz, baby green peas all snug in their pods, tangerines, Krispy Kremes, and barley. The protein in steak helps your body rebuild muscle tissue and repair owwies. The B vitamins in peas may help protect you against heart attacks and reduce stress. Tangerines have vitamin C, to keep you from getting a painful case of scurvy and losing your teeth. Barley is full of fiber and has selenium, which is essential but only in very small amounts. Rocky Snyder recommends eating a variety of foods, just as he recommends a variety of forms of movement. I didn't ask him about Krispy Kremes, though I suspect he doesn't eat them.

When your muscles contract, which is the only way they know how to generate movement, the energy for it comes from a superpowered molecule called adenosine triphosphate, or ATP. ATP functions as the main energy-transferring mechanism within your cells. Usually it needs glucose. Glucose is produced in complicated processes that start with enzymes in your saliva, carry on in your pancreas, and end up in your small intestine, which uses an enzyme to split the slightly more complex sugar molecules down into glucose. Then the bloodstream sends the glucose up into your liver, which acts kind of like a storage tank and glucose dispenser to your cells.

Obviously I have no career ahead of me in biochemistry. But isn't this stuff amazing? The sheer number of chemicals that have to act and react, catalyze and assemble, just so you can get off the couch, is astonishing. And we haven't even talked about the role of creatine or bile, or any other lovely substances that make the getting off the couch happen. Getting off the couch, in and of itself, is a delightful miracle.

The next time you're thinking that your body sucks, remember all the miracles your stomach and liver and cells perform to get you some sugar, and take a moment to appreciate the breathtakingly complex systems that make that body do everything that it does. And then go do something with it.

THE LOWDOWN: MAKING THE WORDS REAL

If you, like me, are attracted to the rebellious idea of fueling your workout with donuts but find that a raised glazed before your morning run makes you hurl, then you've got some options. There are lots of ways to get sugar into your body to prep yourself to move around. This is especially important right after you get up, when your blood glucose is at its lowest, or before and during an extra-long session of moving about.

You can try commercial preparations such as energy gels, which are formulated to blast usable sugars through your stomach, over to the liver, and into your bloodstream at frightening speed. Gels come with brand names like GU (yes, really), PowerGel, Clif Shot, Hammer Gel, Carb-BOOM, and the like. If you have a frosting-lickin' sweet tooth, you'll probably find a gel that you tolerate well and look forward to sucking down. There are also commercially available pre-workout drinks, or you could slug down a can of Ensure or some drinkable yogurt, if you prefer a liquid boost.

If you prefer solid food, it's tricky to find the balance between usable sugars, bulk, and quick digestibility. The banana is an old standby that works for a lot of people, since it is easily converted into pure energy. Some like peanut butter and jelly sandwiches. Yogurt can work too. You probably want to avoid foods with lots of fat, which can make you real queasy, or lots of fiber, which can turn your morning or evening exercise session into a painful and undignified search for the nearest public restroom. Experiment until you find something that allows you to move without feeling bloated or gassy, but still gives you enough sugar to fight the shakes.

22

AVOID CHAFING AT ALL COSTS

FEW THINGS ARE more essential to your happiness as an imperfect athlete than ensuring that your body does not chafe against itself or against other objects. Chafing hurts—a lot. When your thighs are rubbing together to create fiery agony, or your bra strap is cutting into your shoulder like a chainsaw, you can't focus on the essentials of athleticism. You're not having fun, you're not feeling focused or relaxed, and you're probably feeling self-conscious about the fact that the interaction of your imperfect body and your imperfect athletic equipment is causing you such intense yet ridiculous pain. Lest you think I'm exaggerating about the ill effects of chafing, let me just point out that three-time cycling world champion Oscar Freire missed a year of his career due to recurring saddle sores. He eventually needed surgery on what one colleague tactfully referred to as his "undercarriage." Chafing is no joke.

Common places for chafing include the inner thighs, the bra strap area, the inner part of the arm where it may rub up against

117

the torso, and, of course, any part of your anatomy that repeatedly contacts the saddle of a bicycle.

Avoiding chafing is all about making sure that things fit, that they flow freely, that you are not inhibited or held back by your clothing or your gear. It's about minimizing friction. As any physicist will tell you, friction is the single biggest impediment to the continuation of motion, and that is just as true for us as it is for tiny molecules. Chafing is about repetitive friction. The amount of rubbing caused by one step in shorts that ride up on the thigh is laughably small, but when you repeat that 10,000 times, you can end up with a raw, bleeding mess in a really sensitive spot. So how do you minimize friction? Three words: fabric, fit, and lubrication.

Choice of fabric will depend on your sport and your personal preference. Just remember to keep cotton away from your body until you have come to a complete stop on the couch. Cotton, remember, absorbs moisture, gets heavy, and becomes a garden of chafing. Even cotton/Lycra blends are chafe prone if you exercise hard or have any bulges. (Go back and review Chapter 9.) Look for materials that are lightweight and kind of slick, so that your moving parts will slide against each other with little resistance. I always go for the maximum amount of shininess in running tights. It keeps my thighs happy when they encounter each other for the minimum possible time during each stride.

An aside about bicycling. For bike shorts, stretchiness is very important. Look for shorts where the chamois (the padding) also stretches, if possible. This goes a long way toward reducing friction between your legs and the saddle. And if you're a new cyclist, you may be tempted to get the biggest, plumpest, gel-filled chamois you can find to minimize the anticipated discomfort to your rear end. This may be a strategic error. You are basically putting more stuff down there that can get in the way of your movement, and that can cause friction rather than relieving it. Probably better to approach rear-end comfort on a bike by (1) working with your local bike store to make sure the bike fits you properly, (2) gradually, gradually increasing your time in the saddle so that your butt has time to get properly acclimated, (3) spending more money than you would think reasonable on two really good pairs of shorts, and (4) using plenty of lubrication (more on this subject later).

Fit can be a sticking point for a lot of people because it encourages the scourge of self-consciousness to raise its ugly head. Go back and review Chapter 1 and then seek out athletic wear that will fit tightly over the parts most likely to chafe. For me, wide bra straps, long bicycle-cut shorts, and fitted sleeves are essential to a comfortable workout ensemble. Make sure the crotch doesn't sag and the waistband doesn't bind. Make sure the bra is tight (but not cutting into you) rather than loose.

Also, look carefully at the placement of seams and trim when you're considering a new garment. That piece of orange piping on the sleeve may look slick, but will it feel slick when it brushes between your upper arm and your torso for the 5,000th time? When I was training for my marathon, I obsessed over fabric and fit. My longer training runs revealed chafing potential in clothing I had previously considered frictionless. I ended up finding a pair of triathlon shorts that had a pleasing slickness along the inner thighs, being made of a very quick-drying blend of materials. They also had a minimal fleece pad for cycling, but I didn't even notice it while running. I paired the shorts with a white running T-shirt that fit snugly around the upper arms. I was out on that marathon course for over seven hours, and I can proudly say that there was no chafing anywhere above my ankles.

This brings us to the feet. Chafing there usually involves blisters, but sometimes your shoe can dig out a little chunk of flesh which skips the blister stage and goes right to the bleeding. The fit of your shoes, as discussed in Chapter 11, and the fabric of your socks are key to avoiding blisters and hot spots. Sometimes you may be tempted to go sockless on a hot day or during a triathlon. Beware. You're just asking for that little chunk of flesh to be dug out of the arch of your foot or the side of your little toe. The pain from such an injury is ridiculous, especially when you sweat salt into the place where the flesh used to be.

Lubrication is in some ways the most valuable weapon in your antichafing arsenal. You wouldn't run your car without oil, and neither should you venture out on a long workout without some antifriction substance applied to your personal danger zones. My danger zones are the inner thighs, right up to that critical junction of leg with trunk; the area under the chest strap of my sports bra, and the insides of my upper arms. I tend to use BodyGlide for lighter efforts, since it comes in a handy stick and doesn't feel too heavy and greasy. For my marathon, I applied BodyGlide and Vaseline most everywhere, including my feet, and for extra long bike rides, I use a mixture of Vaseline and antibiotic ointment with pain reliever, applied liberally right up to the lower butt cheeks. Whatever lube you use, apply it with a heavy hand and a light heart. Don't get grossed out by lubrication. It's your friend. Once you start working up a good sweat, you won't even notice it's there except by the absence of burning and painful rubbing sensations.

Greased up and snugly encased in technical fabrics, you can go out and cavort to your heart's content, liberated from friction and fear. So what are you waiting for?

23

EAT SOME CHOCOLATE

MY DAY JOB has few perks, but one of them is the proximity of the Scharffen Berger chocolate factory in Berkeley, California. Fortunately my office is far enough away from this temple of earthly delight that I can't smell the tantalizing aroma of the world's finest cacao beans being roasted to perfection; otherwise I'd go mad. A few months ago, though, I joined a group of my coworkers for a tour of the Scharffen Berger plant, and as soon as we got into the parking lot, I felt like I'd died and gone to heaven. It smelled like a Roald Dahl–inspired nirvana. I seriously considered running to the main office and begging them to let me work there as anything, anything at all.

The tour was fascinating. I was delighted to discover that dark chocolate has something like three times as many flavor-influencing organic compounds as red wine. As part of the tour, we tasted roasted cacao nibs, which have such an astounding variety of flavors that the idea of adding sugar seems almost superfluous. At the end of the afternoon I was convinced that there is no point in eating cheap commercial chocolate ever again.

Eating chocolate judiciously will help keep you from obsessing over eating "virtuously" as you engage in your athletic endeavors. Some people go overboard once they take up a new regimen of physical activity.

Oh, and for heaven's sake, please don't justify eating dark chocolate with the trendy information that dark chocolate is full of antioxidants. You do not need a "healthy" excuse to eat great chocolate. Great chocolate is its own justification. Period.

For another thing, eating a really wonderful piece of chocolate is an incredible physical sensation. I make no claims to having a superfine palate, but letting a small bite of the intense dark velvet melt on your tongue, resisting the urge to chew, trying to pick out hints of coffee, earth, wine, malt, berries, stout, and other flavors within the overwhelming surge of chocolate is mind-blowing. It focuses your whole being on the present moment and the sumptuous satisfaction that can result in the interaction between your marvelously complex body and the marvelously complex world around it. And you can do it in public too.

Taking a few moments to savor the nearly infinite depth and richness of great chocolate enhances your appreciation of life. It heightens your senses and makes you wonder at the possibilities inherent in the world around you. After you have enjoyed the chocolate right down to the last echo of the last subtle, bitter aftertaste, stop and think about the process that made that chocolate possible, and you will be awed all over again.

You can't eat cacao straight off the tree. It's either poisonous or very, very icky, I forget which. Maybe both. The cacao seeds (or "beans") have to be extracted from their pods, skillfully fermented for a period of days, then dried at just the right moment. Miss one step along the way, and you end up with inedible lumps.

Of course, the same sense of wonder can be conjured up around a number of edibles and drinkables. Wine, of course, but also cheese, and even a simple loaf of bread. I've been known to drift off into raptures over each.

Maybe it's a stretch to say that chocolate making parallels your striving toward athleticism, but indulge me. The cacao pod grows wild in the hot, humid forests of the tropics. It is a natural phenomenon, as are you, growing only slightly wild in the cities or suburbs of North America or wherever you happen to be. Like the cacao pod, you are a magnificent manifestation of the natural world. But in order to reach your full potential as a human being and as an athlete, you, like the cacao pod, need to undergo a number of painstaking, time-consuming processes. You need to be tended lovingly by family and friends for your emotional and social development. You need to be educated enough to function in your society, and you need to be cultivated physically in order to develop full energy and health.

But without the essential nature of the cacao pod, the innate structure that allows its seeds to contain hundreds of flavor-bearing chemicals, all those painstaking processes are futile. The same goes for you. Your complexity, your greatness as a human being, your physical ability, yes, your athleticism, all are packed tightly into your DNA, just waiting for the right processing to turn you into the rich, full-flavored, deeply satisfying phenomenon that you can be.

So every bite of good chocolate should remind you of the miracle of molding unlikely raw material into something as perfect as it can possibly be. It is a tasty metaphor for you, and all that you are in the process of becoming. So there.

TAKE A NAP

I **NEVER USED** to be big on naps. It wasn't until I got a way down the road to my imperfect athleticism that I began to embrace the concept of napping. More accurately, I guess, napping began to embrace me. I think it was after my second triathlon, which was a lot longer and harder than the first one. I got home, tossed my filthy gear on the patio, showered extensively, scarfed a chicken burrito, and hit my brick-red recliner, the spiritual heir to my dad's harvest-gold nap machine. I intended to watch the Giants game, but somewhere around the third inning, I began sinking into oblivion. And it was nice. Very, very nice. Floating away on fluffy clouds of slumber type of nice.

Since that seminal nap, I have napped after most, though not all, of my major races. In fact, I've built it into my race-day schedule. Pack. Drive. Set up. Race. Drink fluids. Pack. Drive. Buy burrito. Sit in recliner. Turn on sports event. Sink gradually into somnolent bliss. Drool on myself.

Yeah, the nap was just a nap. People take them all the time. But what it brought home to me was that unbreakable connection between effort and recovery, and that full recovery doesn't take place when your eyes are open. Sleeping is what fixes your body when you expend a massive store of your available energy. It also fixes you over the long term, when you expend physical and mental energy on a consistent basis.

When you're asleep, your pituitary gland, a pea-size unit at the base of your brain, releases human growth hormone (HGH). This chemical is not the fountain of youth, no matter what the spam in your inbox may proclaim. But it is a truly remarkable compound, the exact functions of which I am unqualified to explain. But let me give it a shot anyway. It helps to balance your body's protein supply. When you exercise, the bod breaks down proteins, and HGH controls other hormones that signal the body to synthesize new proteins. HGH is in charge, in a delegating CEO kind of way, of rebuilding bone and producing collagen, the primordial goo that helps build new tissue. It also seems to be involved in regulating how you metabolize fat. The point is that getting HGH into your system is a good thing, as long as you produce it yourself; no magic pills.

The pituitary produces surges of HGH throughout the day, but the biggest one happens while you sleep. Another thing that stimulates the production of HGH is exercise. This is great, since you are on the yellow brick trail to imperfect athleticism, and your plans include plenty of exercise. But remember, exercise breaks down protein and causes little traumas to your connective tissue. You need more HGH to help fix them, so make sure that you get enough sleep at night. But does napping help you get more HGH pumping from your tiny little pituitary?

A scholarly article I read on PubMed gave the results of an experiment where people took morning or afternoon naps. Sure enough, napping seemed to raise the level of HGH released in the subjects' brains, with afternoon napping raising HGH more than morning napping. The gist of the research is that HGH gets produced during a phase of sleep called slow-wave sleep, which doesn't get as much press as REM sleep but is extremely useful. It's very deep sleep, very hard to wake up from, and it's the kind your body craves most if you're deprived of sleep. So when you go down for a hard nap, where waking up is like swimming to the surface from deep in the ocean, you're getting some slow-wave, HGH sleep.

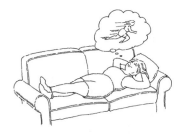

But besides all the scientific benefits of napping, you have to give proper respect to the bliss factor. Napping is part of the fun of training and competing. It's a wonderful reward for your hard work; it's totally free, and now that you know about HGH, you can explain to your significant other that the nap is not a symptom of laziness but an integral part of your imperfectly athletic regimen. Plus, when you're napping, you can't be forced or guilt-tripped into yard work, vacuuming the living room, or doing laundry. You're busy recovering.

You don't have to race to deserve an afternoon nap. A long, tiring workout will give you a perfect rationale for seizing the snoozy moment. A nice training session that leaves you feeling pleasantly leaden and the ingestion of some tasty carbohydrates are all the preparation you need. Add a comfy couch or La-Z-Gal recliner, a television, and maybe a towel to catch any drooly droplets, and you are set.

If you don't happen to have a long training session under your belt but you have the carbs and the recliner and you find your eyelids drooping, I say go ahead and take a nap. You probably need it. You'll get a little boost of HGH, and you'll have a little bliss in the bank for next time you need extra fortitude.

Take a nap. For recovery or for fun. It's an essential, if perhaps counterintuitive, element of kicking butt. Even more important, it's an essential part of your overall health and happiness.

25

ESCHEW DIETS

I'M NOT A fan of diets. They don't work and they feed dangerous illusions. I have gained and lost hundreds of pounds, starting in my early teens, and here I am again at 250 pounds, plus or minus a cheeseburger or two. I don't even remember my first diet. It might have been Dr. Atkins's low-carb craziness, or I might have joined my mom's Weight Watchers program.

The same mental skills that that served me in good stead as an endurance athlete worked to my advantage as a child dieter. I had the ability to focus on a task, repeat certain specified activities, and endure discomfort or exert effort in pursuit of my objective. I was motivated by the idea of measurable achievement, perhaps even more by praise, sometimes even by money. At least once during my dieting career Mom paid me a dollar for every pound I lost.

Besides early Weight Watchers and something to do with grapefruit, there was a version of the cabbage soup diet, which has been around for many years. A cool book called *Paradox of Plenty* by Harvey Levenstein includes a whole bunch of stuff about fad diets during the height of the Great Depression.

Pleasingly plump went out in the 1920s, and by the 1930s a ca-
bal of doctors and dietitians were spreading the word that excess weight, rather than being an enviable mark of affluence,
might be bad for your health. So the decade that I associate
with soup kitchens, bread riots, and scavengers in the garbage
dump was actually marked by a wave of diet fads. Women of the
upper and middle classes were embracing a variety of weight
loss schemes that might have a familiar ring to modern dieters.
Never eat proteins and carbohydrates at the same time? It's the
1930s Hay diet, named for Dr. William Hay. The United Fruit
Company, known for bringing the phrase "banana republic" to
linguistic prominence, promoted a diet of skim milk and—
surprise—bananas! An unfashionably plump young miss in the
1930s could attempt to "burn up ugly fat" with the pineapple
and lamb chop diet, the potato and buttermilk diet, or the raw
tomato and hard-boiled egg diet. You could eat "slo-baked"
Wonder Bread, which purported to give you a quick burst of energy so you could "diet with a smile." Gad.

We don't study our national dieting history, so we're con-
demned to repeat it. I tried Nutri-System and I tried fasting. I
tried macrobiotic combinations of brown rice, steamed vegetables, and tofu. I even tried Atkins the second time around. But
dieting doesn't work. We all know it doesn't work, but we sucker
ourselves into it time and time again.

Why do we continue to delude ourselves? I think the core of
the delusion is "I'll just lose ten pounds, then I'll eat moderately
for a while, then I'll do the diet again and lose ten more
pounds." The rub is that we chronic dieters don't know how to
eat moderately. We only know how to overeat and undereat. Especially the former. And the undereating awakens a deep-seated

physiological appetite for things like fats and sugar, highly caloric fuels that can stave off the famine that our bodies think is coming. So when we lose the ten pounds, or before then if the cravings get too strong, we don't just go back to how we were eating before the diet; we eat both with the millennia-old survival instincts and with the desire for long-denied gratification of the forbidden food. It's a combination of our digestive/metabolic biochemistry urging us to up our calorie intake and our brain chemistry going, "I *want* it!" The stress of being underfed raises the brain's production of dopamine, which drives goal-seeking activity. And our goal-seeking activity is focused on the donut.

Humans aren't built to diet. We're built to pursue scarce food supplies. When rich food is available, we're engineered to eat as much of it as we can, to binge, in effect. But throughout human history, food supplies have rarely been so abundant as to enable us to build up much surplus fat before we have to work it off again through hunting, gathering, farming, or travel, or lose it through a dry season or a long winter. The threat of famine has been the driving force behind the evolution of our bodies' appetites and eating patterns for thousands and thousands of years.

But starting in the twentieth century, for most people in America, food became overabundant. We can eat as much as we want, and way more than we need. The cheapest food is the fattiest, sugariest, or saltiest stuff around, all designed to speak to the cravings shaped by the Serengeti. We try to fight the cravings with every weapon we can think of, and the fad diet is one of those weapons.

We early-twenty-first century Americans have a lot of cultural assumptions around the phrase "diet and exercise," and I

invite you to scrutinize your own assumptions carefully. Sub-
jecting yourself to cabbage soup and skim milk, just like sub-
jecting yourself to exercise you don't enjoy, is focusing on the
negatives about your body, rather than the magical things it
can do. For more on movement for its own sake versus movement for weight loss, see Chapter 39.

26

FIND A DOCTOR WHO LISTENS

EXCESS WEIGHT HAS been linked to increased risk of some very nasty things. I am still petrified by a 2004 issue of *Newsweek* that I keep stashed in my research materials box. Blown up to a gazillion times life size, a hideous, spherical fat cell looms in digitally enhanced color, the monster in a cheesy science fiction movie. "When Fat Cells ATTACK," the headline blares. I read, horrified, about how my overstuffed fat cells, especially the ones around my voluminous belly, are little engines of destruction inside my body. They're leading to chronic inflammatory response, creating fertile ground for diabetes, cancer, heart disease, and other illnesses du jour. Yes, the potential for my superfluous weight to cause problems is scary, but that weight is not everything about me. It's not even everything about my body.

Even at 250 pounds, my blood pressure hangs at around 115 over 80, and my resting pulse is about 55 to 65 beats per minute, depending on whether I get to wake up at my own speed or get jolted out of bed by the alarm. At 245 to 255, I competed in a marathon and six triathlons last year, including two pretty challenging Olympic distance courses. That's .91 miles of swimming, 24.8 on the bike, and a brisk 6.2-mile jog to finish it off. I may be slow and I may be fat, but I am an athlete. I've been training for running and triathlon for nearly seven years now, and I understand my body pretty well.

But even if you haven't been training athletically for years on end, you understand your body pretty well. You know your baseline energy level; you know when you're more tired than normal; you know when you feel a little sick; you know when you feel strong and ready for adventure. Doctors are experts in diseases and treatments, but we are experts in the strengths and weaknesses of our bodies, and a good doctor respects our expertise.

I once went to see a doctor about some weird spots on my leg that I thought might be Lyme disease. I had been backpacking, and a few days after I got back, I noticed these red patches. I decided they were spider bites and didn't think of them again until a few days later, when they seemed bigger and redder. At the same time, I was feeling sluggish and achy, sleeping a ton, feeling "off."

The possibility of Lyme disease first drifted across my consciousness in an online discussion of insect bites. I didn't have the typical ring and bull's-eye rash, but some pictures of atypical Lyme rashes looked similar to mine. I read about the early symptoms of Lyme: fatigue, body aches, vague malaise. I also read that the Sierra Nevada is not a hotbed of Lyme, but that cases do occur. We had done some off-trail hiking through thick brush too.

By the time I could get an appointment with a doctor, the blotches were starting to fade, losing their impressive scarlet color and slightly raised appearance. Foreseeing this eventuality, I had taken pictures of them just past their peak. I couldn't get an appointment with my own doctor so I settled for one of the other docs in the practice.

I explained my symptoms, my blotches, my trip in the Sierras, our bushwhacking hikes. I told her that it was unusual for me to feel so tired and draggy, that I was feeling body aches that seemed unrelated to the hiking we had done. The hiking, though strenuous on the first day, had gotten easier. We had acclimatized to the altitude, gained some fitness, and lightened our packs by eating up our food. By the end of the trip I was feeling strong and nimble on my feet.

This doctor, however, thought I was feeling bad because I was fat. "Do you get much exercise?" she inquired. "Because the scale shows that you've gained a lot of weight over the past year, and I think that is a much more probable cause of your fatigue and malaise." I was stunned. What part of "six-day backpacking trip up over not one but two passes higher than 11,000 feet" did she not understand? What part of "I'm a triathlete" did she not hear? My heart began to beat a little harder and I felt a little queasy.

"Um, yeah, I do triathlons? So I exercise five to ten hours a week. I run, bike, or swim almost every day, sometimes twice a day. I know my energy levels, and I know when I'm feeling run down. Why would I feel fine in the mountains when I was exerting myself for hours every day and feel like crap when I come back, if it was all to do with weight gain?"

She was undeterred from her vision of me as an unhealthy person, dragged down so severely by extra poundage that it was a miracle I could get up the stairs to the clinic. "I'd like to run some blood tests to check out the possibility of diabetes and hypothyroidism, either of which I think are far more likely to be causing your fatigue than Lyme disease." She went on to ask me if I snored, which I had to admit to, and if my husband had noticed me stopping breathing in my sleep. "I think it might be worth doing a comprehensive sleep study on you. Sleep apnea is extremely common among overweight people, and it can lead to serious health consequences."

I was starting to feel really crappy now. Diabetes? Thyroid disease? Sleep apnea? I didn't think I had any of those things, but I didn't really know. Maybe my weight gain over the past couple of years really had brought with it a host of serious and chronic health problems. I left the office with the doctor's injunction to keep from gaining any more weight ringing in my ears. I sat docilely in the lab while my blood was drawn.

It wasn't until I got in my car that I started to get mad. Okay, I'm fat. Okay, I'm fatter this year than I was before. But what gave that (skinny, little) doctor the right to completely disregard my immediate concerns, dismiss my own hard-won knowledge of my body and its fitness, and tell me that the only likely reason I am feeling unwell is that I'm fat? "Fat" does not automatically equal "unwell," just as "old" doesn't mean "stupid." I had been stereotyped in the most egregious way, and I was fuming. But the thing about being fat—it's pretty hard in our culture to argue that it's not important. I called a friend and railed about the humiliation as I choked on tears of pain and rage.

The saddest thing is that Bad Doc really thought she was taking the right approach to my issue. She really thought she was doing the best thing for me by dismissing my observations and intelligence, criticizing me for my weight gain, and ordering tests for maladies I did not have.

A week or so after my encounter with Bad Doc, I made an appointment with my regular doc. I wanted to go over my test results with her and also get her opinion on the whole Lyme thing. Even though Good Doc told me the same thing about the unlikelihood of having Lyme, the experience was completely different in every other way. Good Doc listened to me, challenged my hypothesis about leg blotches and body aches as an intelligent adult would with another intelligent adult, commented that I knew my body well, and offered other possible solutions for what ailed me. She saw me, not just my fat.

It's not a bad idea to get tests for common and insidious chronic diseases, certainly, if you are carrying a lot of weight or haven't exercised in a long time, or ever. Diabetes is serious. If you have a freaky thyroid, it can be a big problem. You want to know if your blood pressure is high or if you have sleep apnea. Good Doc tells me that your "sleep partner" will almost inevitably report those periods when you stop breathing and then start again with a scary noise. If you don't have a sleep partner, try road-tripping with a light-sleeping friend for a few days and sharing a room. But being overweight or a few decades past your twenties, or having a long history as a couch potato—nothing gives a doctor the right to belittle your knowledge of your body or speak to you in a condescending manner. It's just not cool.

So if you have a doctor who can't see past your layer of fat—or your age or your whatever—change doctors. Even in this age of seven-minute doctor-patient encounters, there are still doctors out there who will treat you as a responsible partner in your own health. It can be hard to trust yourself when the intimidating white coat intones his or her professional opinion. But if you have a serious issue and the doctor won't listen, it's perfectly acceptable to talk back. You don't have to be docile just because your body is not perfect. Do research, find articles, and persist until you get the answers you need. Maybe you'll be wrong, as I was about Lyme disease, but you'll be a participant in your own health care, not just a spectator.

And pay attention to your body, gather data on it so you can speak confidently about what is and is not normal for you. We'll talk more about the joys of data in Chapter 38, but getting reliable information can be as simple as just paying attention to daily good feelings or aches and pains. As a culture, we're pretty much conditioned to be out of tune with our bodies, to ignore the pain in the neck from driving, the stiffness from sitting, the pain in the wrist from keyboarding. Don't ignore it any more.

You're an athlete, and you know your body. Make sure your doctor knows you know.

MIND THE IBUPROFEN

THE FAVORITE OF many endurance athletes and weekend
warriors worldwide, "vitamin I" is consumed in mass quantities by people who are getting back into exercise; who are
training long and hard for some gruel fest like an Ironman or an
AIDS ride; or who have some nagging injury they just want to
get calmed down.

Ibuprofen has relieved pain and inflammation for millions of
people. It works, scientists believe, by controlling the body's
synthesis of a hormone called prostaglandin, which affects the
inflammatory response to injury, stress, or injury. Some triathletes tape the little brown pills to their bikes so they can take
them as they ride. For people who tolerate vitamin I well, it's
pretty much a miracle drug.

But ibuprofen can play havoc with the lining of your stomach and intestines. You can get a bleeding ulcer or a hole in
your innards with no warning. I can't take even one ibuprofen
without feeling searing gastrointestinal pain. But even people
who feel like they tolerate it just fine can end up with serious
nastiness in the stomach.

Ibuprofen isn't the only painkiller that can mess you up, of course. Old-fashioned aspirin can make your stomach bleed, and a lot of people who can't take aspirin take IbuP like candy. Acetaminophen, more commonly known as Tylenol, is easier on the stomach, but it can cause liver damage if you take too much of it.

I'm not writing this as a screed against immensely popular and useful medications that pose little risk if used sparingly and occasionally. A little painkiller now and then is just the ticket. After a very tough workout or a race, certainly if you have a traumatic injury like a sprained ankle or banged-up knee, your over-the-counter painkiller is exactly what you need. You want to reduce inflammation as much as possible. So ice whatever part of your body hurts and take a little something from the drugstore, preferably with some food to protect your stomach.

But beware if you find yourself popping painkillers as a matter of habit. Your back hurts every morning, so you take some. You have to take some after every run because your heel hurts. Nagging shoulder or neck or calf or hip pain. All that stuff. You're busy, you're sore, but you don't hurt bad enough to go to the doctor so you pop some ibuprofen/aspirin/acetaminophen and you're good to go another day.

If that's you, or if it starts happening to you down the road, stop. Figure out how long you've been in pain and, first of all, get some rest. Quit doing the things that make you hurt and find some other things that don't aggravate the pain. If the pain doesn't go away, refer to Chapter 43 and go get some help. Get a referral for physical therapy; get ultrasound, or at least get advice from a doctor. If your doctor's advice doesn't work, go back. Don't be afraid to look around for a doctor with greater expertise or a different perspective. Massage therapists who are qualified to do sports massage and deep tissue work can perform small miracles on nagging injuries. Sometimes you need to see a specialist in foot issues or sports medicine to figure out what's going on. Persist. Don't let minor pain escalate into a big problem or affect other parts of your anatomy. A problem in your knee might actually be emanating from your hip, and if you don't get that core issue fixed you may end up with a bad back. You compensate for weakness or strain in one part of your body by overusing another part, and the domino effect can take you out of commission for a long time. Even if you don't get a domino effect, you can still aggravate your initial injury if you are taking ibuprofen or other painkillers like candy.

So you can take your Advil or your Tylenol or your Bayer for occasional soreness, but when the pain becomes constant, that's a warning. Monitor your consumption of those little pills and don't let twinges and tweaks turn into something chronic or serious. Being an athlete, even—or especially—an imperfect athlete, means listening attentively to your body. Pain is the most obvious communication from your body that things are not as they should be. It's not a genteel Jeevesian, "If I might be so bold as to make a suggestion, sir, this shooting pain in my knee could perhaps be a sign of an incipient injury to the iliotibial band." It's more like a New York cabbie in heavy traffic: YO! Ya freakin' MORON! What kind of dumbass move is THAT!" So listen up.

SECTION IV

NINE TIPS FOR DEALING WITH THE WORLD YOU LIVE IN

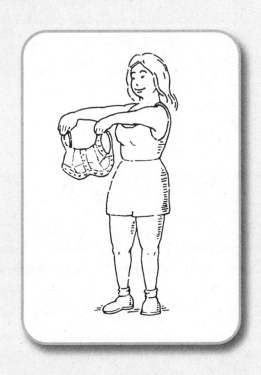

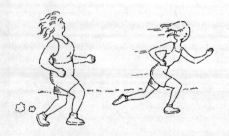

BE SELFISH

J UST BECAUSE YOU'RE working to practice compassion toward yourself and others doesn't mean you can't be selfish.
Not selfish in a "give me all the mashed potatoes right now"
kind of way, but selfish in a way that enables you to dedicate
regular time to your athletic goals. The best technique for exercising selfishness involves saying no to your job whenever possible (see Chapter 29) and going for a bike ride or grabbing
your kayak for a quick paddle before the sun goes down. I mean,
do your job, but don't volunteer to stay late to prepare the report on the implications of the unexpected fourth-quarter up-
swing in global ferret farming as it relates to standards-based
educational policy in rural Nebraska. Let someone else do the
dirty work this time.

Saying no to work is relatively easy. Just keep practicing.
(Then, when you get fired, you'll have loads of time to work
out.) But for a lot of people, it's way harder to tell a boyfriend,
girlfriend, spouse, or kids that they're going to have fend for
themselves on Monday and Wednesday evenings so that you
can go to your spin class. You're already not spending enough

quality time with these important people in your life, and now you want to take off and leave them in a lonely haze of frozen dinners and reruns of *American Chopper*. You are a Bad Person, you figure. And so you stay home instead, and you get all grouchy and physically stiff and sore from not working out. Which is great for your relationship with your loved ones, obviously.

Here's my rationale for spending slightly less time with your family in favor of more time pursuing your dreams of improved athleticism. Moving your body more and becoming happier with your more mobile body makes you a Better Person. And wouldn't your family rather spend three hours a night with a Better Person than four and a half hours with a Grumpy Person who feels crappy about her increasingly immobile body? Exercise, as any doctor, personal trainer, or moderately literate person who reads *Time* magazine knows, relieves stress. Would your boyfriend, girlfriend, or roommate not prefer to see you in a happy, endorphin-filled, unstressed state than in your post-office, postcommute, ready-to-pitch-a-hissy-fit-of-gargantuan-proportions weekday evening mood? To me, this seems like a great big "duh."

When I get home from a day so long and exhausting that I can't face going out and moving my body at all, the impact on my sweet and patient husband is far more negative than if I get home even later, having spent a happy hour sweating, grunting, breathing hard, and finishing it up with ten blissful minutes in a turbo-powered Jacuzzi. When I come home from work and don't exercise, I start complaining vociferously. I complain about traffic, unresponsive clients, state and county bureaucracies, my tired back, my aching head, and my lack of energy. But when I exercise, all but the most grievous of my daily complaints evaporate in the rhythm of my breathing and the pumping of my legs, or the regular splash and burble of my stately progress through the pool. I come home relaxed and pleasantly fatigued, smelling faintly of chlorine or not so faintly of sweat if I've been outside rather than at the gym. I take a shower and then give Tim a smacky-smack mwah-mwah kiss and a big hug, and I hardly complain at all. A good session of moving my body around makes me feel so happy I could hug anyone who happened to be in the house when I got home. (Look out, cable guys!)

Sometimes you have to bail on brunch with your girlfriends at your favorite purveyor of eggs Benedict in favor of your long bike ride and your nap. Or you turn down happy hour with the work buds to do your core strength and flexibility class. You may hear snarky remarks about how you're becoming holier than thou, or an unbalanced fitness addict, or how you're just no fun anymore. These may not be your truest friends. You may blow them off with a clear conscience if you think they're just defensive about their own persistent immobility or body-hating issues. But if you examine their personalities, the history of your relationship, and their motivation for making these re-marks, and you still think they are true and loyal, then it's time to think deeply. Same goes for your family's griping. Are you becoming obnoxious? Are you turning into an exercise snob? Are you bragging incessantly about how much stronger you are and how much better you feel, with the (probably) inadvertent effect of making them feel bad? Are you getting obsessive, freaking out if you miss even one scheduled workout?

If so, lower your volume and intensity, at least externally. In-ternally, keep braggin' on your bad self just as loud and fre-quently as you possibly can. Try being inconsistent for once (see Chapter 16).

However you work it, keep moving your body, even if it inconveniences someone else's schedule once in a while. Fight anyone who tries to take that away from you. Maybe fight nicely, with kindness and diplomacy rather than carpet bombing, but fight anyway. Kick ass on your own behalf. You deserve it.

THE LOWDOWN: MAKING THE WORDS REAL

How can you get into the habit of being productively selfish—looking out for your athleticism without alienating those who help make your life possible?

Put the time in your calendar. Mark it "private appointment" if you want to, so that your coworkers can't schedule stupid meetings over it.

Invite people along. Maybe they shudder at the thought of going for a session of vigorous CrossFit with you, but at least they know you value their company. Who knows, maybe somebody will actually try your activity of choice and thank you for it. But don't hold your breath.

Bribe them. Buy them gifts large and small so they don't complain about your not being there. The catch here is you can't already be bribing your loved ones to forgive your absences; otherwise this additional campaign to win their affection will lose its impact. But a little material love here or there never hurt anyone, right?

Schedule them in, too. This may seem like a "duh," but don't forget it in your excitement over being a new or returning athlete. One very disciplined triathlete would get up and do his whole Saturday workout early in the morning, giving up his one opportunity to sleep in, so he could be done by noon and spend the rest of the day with his wife and two kids.

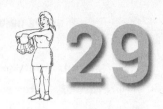

WORK LESS
(AT YOUR JOB)

THE BOOK-BUYING world being what it is, a lot of you, my dear readers, will be overeducated professionals who spend the majority of their waking hours at their desk and in their car and think, "Wow, I really need to get more exercise." I myself am an overeducated semiprofessional type, and on a typical day I drive for two and a half hours, sit at a computer or in meetings for eight to eight and three-quarters hours, and spend about a half-hour getting into and out of my work clothes. I allocate about twenty-five minutes to showering, basic hygiene (no makeup, no blow-dryer), and dressing, and about ten minutes goes to flinging off my work clothes the instant I get through the door and searching out my softest sweatshirt and my velour lounge pants.

If we add up those hours, which may be a little light on the actual work (by the standards of the average overachieving American) but just over twice the national average commute time, we end up with ten and three-quarters to eleven and three-quarters hours of each day dedicated to work and the logistics of work. This is probably somewhere in your range too. Another seven and a half to eight and a half hours are dedicated to sleeping and the logistics of getting ready for sleep: ascertaining whereabouts of cats, dogs, kids, turning off lights and appliances, rudimentary evening toilette, picking out tomorrow's outfit, kissing husband goodnight. Add an hour for dinner and dishes and an hour of quality television (everything I understand about science I learned from *Mythbusters*) or quality time with the kids, and we're up to around twenty-two hours out of most weekdays that are not available for exercising. You could sleep less. A lot of people do. But I am not a person who functions well on short rations of sleep and I bet you don't either.

Back to those hours that are available for exercising. If we look at them closely, even on the days where everything takes a little longer—the commute is suckier, the meetings don't end on time, and the dishes are particularly crusty—there may still be an hour available to me for exercise.

The key is figuring out where that hour is so that you can become the imperfect athlete of your dreams.

First, figure out your schedule, Monday through Sunday. I start with Monday because it's a common convention in training calendars. The tendency is to put your longer, harder workouts on Saturday or Sunday to finish out the week and make Monday a rest day. Then you build up again toward the weekend.

Block out the all the time: getting up and getting ready for your day, getting your offspring ready, feeding your whiny pets, your commute, your work, your other commute, your evening responsibilities. Schedule your sleep. Please do not make the mistake of scheduling less sleep in order to become an imperfect athlete. As you up your activity levels, you will need more

Aspiring Athlete's Sample Workday Schedule (for Nonmorning Person)	
6:15–6:30 A.M.	Stumble from bed; shower, rudimentary toilette.
6:30–6:40 A.M.	Dress in simple outfit laid out the night before.
6:35–6:37 A.M.	Feed whiny pet.
6:37–6:44 A.M.	Dry hair.
6:45–6:47 A.M.	Grab lunch laid out the night before, take morning pills.
6:47–7:30 A.M.	Wake kids, if any. Feed them. Clothe them.
7:30–7:45 A.M.	Kids to school.
7:45–8:30 A.M.	Commute to work. Combine with drinking water, listening to audiobook.
8:35 A.M.–4:45 P.M.	Day job. Eat healthy yet quick breakfast and lunch so you can leave early. Prioritize time so as not to get trapped in office doing bits and pieces.
4:48–5:40 P.M.	Drive home. Curse traffic. Get kids from afterschool program.
5:40–5:50 P.M.	Recover from drive. Kiss husband. Look at mail, ignore bills.
5:50–6:00 P.M.	Get out of work clothes and into workout clothes.
6:00–6:10 P.M.	Give kids a snack to shut them up.
6:10–7:00 P.M.	Ride bike or run or do a gym thing. Enjoy feeling of moving muscles.
7:00–7:15 P.M.	Divest self of now sweaty cycling clothes, stretch.
7:15–7:25 P.M.	Very quick shower.
7:25–7:50 P.M.	Eat dinner (thanks, hubby).
7:50–9:00 P.M.	Help kids with homework; do other parental stuff.
9:00–9:30 P.M.	Get kids to bed.
9:30–9:45 P.M.	"Your time!" Enjoy all fifteen minutes of it.
9:45–10:10 P.M.	Do dishes, lay out lunch(es).
10:10–10:20 P.M.	Lay out tomorrow's clothes, very rudimentary evening toilette.
10:20–10:40 P.M.	Read mystery novel (not too enthralling).
10:41 P.M.–6:15 A.M.	Sleep.

sleep. Maybe not right away, as you start slow and easy, with twenty-or thirty-minute sessions. But as you start to put out more effort on a regular basis, your body is going to need those Zs. We'll return to this later, but trust me now: your sleep is one of the most important parts of getting fit. Your bod cannot recover sufficiently from one ass-kicking session to kick ass again the next time if you're short on sleep.

If you're not used to doing this, your first look at your hour-by-hour schedule may send you into a panic attack. How are you going to do everything (not to mention all those other things you're not doing but should be doing)?

Breathe. Relax. You'll just have to give some things up. I myself have given up cooking, most housecleaning, and running all but the most essential errands. I have not been to the dry cleaner in two years. Yeah, the house is a little dirtier and my wardrobe is less spiffy than it might otherwise be, but last year I did a marathon, a two-day relay race, and six triathlons. I also put in eight hundred miles on my bike in the past three and a half months of the year. Pare down to the bare minimum. If you have your kids sleep in the clothes they're going to wear to school the next day and you still can't find time to move your body about, you might want to examine whether having fun moving your body about is the kind of fun you most want to have. Maybe you don't.

Alternatively, see if you can give up some work. Especially if you're a salary slave. I know this reeks of subversiveness, possibly even communism, but I think that putting in endless hours on the treadmill of corporate America does not always enhance your quality of life. You put in your sixty-hour weeks, you live on coffee and vending machine food, and then your company merges with some multinational megacorporation and there you are, sacrificed to economies of scale and shareholder value. Even if you own your own business and do work that you love, it's bad news to get so far out of balance that you can't go for a thirty-minute jog a couple of times during the work week.

Perhaps not surprisingly, most of the research I found on the negative impact of getting your job out of whack with your life was from other countries: Australia, New Zealand, the United Kingdom, Canada. The Canadian public-private partnership JobQuality.ca reports that people who feel overloaded at work are less likely to feel healthy and more likely to feel depressed and/or stressed, by a pretty large margin. And are those overloaded people out moving their bodies in a joyful way? Probably not. This seems like a "duh," but sometimes we lose track of it because we're so darn busy, or we decide that the exercise is not as important.

Making time for physical activity that you enjoy (as opposed to vacuuming or cleaning your gutters) ultimately makes you a better worker. You sleep better, you reduce stress, you have more energy, and you feel better about life. If you are a salary slave, then grow some cojones and leave the office when the clock strikes five. The work will wait—most days. I have to put in some long days at the work desk too. I know how it is.

If you're working an hourly job and you don't have flexibility in when you work and how much you work, you have a tougher row to hoe. Working less might not be an option. And that sucks.

Either way, you have to get creative. If you run right after work, will that help you miss the worst of the commute hours, so you get home only 20 minutes later than you otherwise would have, even after your 30 minute run?

Figure out ways to have more fun, work less, play more. You'll be a better, happier, and more productive person.

THE LOWDOWN: MAKING THE WORDS REAL

How can you squeeze in an exercise session when your life is already squeezed?

Lisa in Chicago runs to work, carrying her clothes (which must be made of miracle fabric) in a tight-fitting backpack and showering at a gym next to her office.

Can you commute on your bike with some travel-worthy knit work clothes in a bag? Can you swim during lunch?

Can you take your kids to the park and run laps around them as they play on the climbing structures?

Can you lift them like weights—pumping babies? Those little dudes are heavy.

Can you cook something on Sunday that can be reheated during the week, thus freeing you for the spin class on Tuesday or a thousand yards in the pool on Wednesday?

Can you enlist your entire family in your quest for butt-kicking fitness? Play two-on-two basketball together by moonlight?

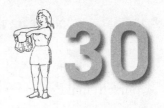

GO ALONE

SOME PEOPLE TELL me they want to train for an event or take up a new sport, but they can't find anyone to do it with them. So they don't do it. Yeah, all right, I know it can be intimidating to walk into a new class or club meeting or join a group bike ride all by yourself. But hey, if you're going to be an athlete (and you are), you are going to face things that are far more intimidating than that. You're going to have to deal with all that sweat, for one thing. I encourage you to muster up your courage and your initiative and just go alone.

Don't use the rationale of not having a training partner or a workout buddy as an excuse to avoid starting your new sport.

Going alone can be good for you. You'll be forced to talk to new people; you'll make new acquaintances, maybe even friends who can mentor you and show you the ropes of your new sport. You may find other newbies who are in the same clueless boat as yourself. You may feel less inhibited by the persona you inhabit with your friends or your significant other, and able to let your inner athlete roar and rant. After all, your new sport friends don't know that you have spent thirty-four years

153

avoiding exercise and that the idea of competing, even with yourself, makes you break out in a rash. It's a fresh start.

Another aspect of going alone is really going alone. Even if you are a social person, exercising can be that rare time for you to be solitary, doing your own thing at your own pace, not interacting with anyone else, save for a quick wave or a nod here and there. You don't need to be completely out of sight or hearing of all other humans; it's more that you can be focused on your workout, your goal for the day, or the weird little thoughts going through your head. You can think about your training and your big athletic dreams, or you can think about nothing. Or you can think about nothing but your breathing or your posture or your rhythm. It's just all about you. And you may like that sometimes.

What about when you're all fired up, trained and ready, and you're going to do your first big event? Your tae kwon do tournament, your outrigger regatta, your 10k run, your triathlon is coming up and your significant other says, ah, honey, I don't want to get up at 6:00 A.M. on a Saturday just to watch you disappear into the distance for an hour or two. What do you do? You go alone. Preferably without getting all guilt-trippy on his or her ass. Ultimately, this athlete business is Your Thing. If hubby or wifey wants to share it with you, great. If he or she wants to come just for the absolutely epic events, great. If not, think about the dozen other ways your dear ones support you: maybe by never making you feel guilty for heading out for a triathlon adventure and leaving him or her at home. Maybe by making dinner or taking care of the housework so that you can train. Maybe by buying you cute socks.

Get in your car, find a car pool, do a road trip. Road trips are fun. Find an event in a quaint part of your state. Every state in the Union has charming areas. So find a fun road race or festival of snowshoeing or canoe trip and get in your car by yourself and go there. Being alone, as many sage persons have observed before me, is not the same thing as being lonely. Being lonely involves unhappiness and being unsatisfied with your own company. Being alone, on the other hand, means that people aren't continually bugging you with inanities or their own taste in music or their ridiculously frequent peeing schedules.

Life is pretty complicated and crowded with people, responsibilities, obligations, traffic, and different media screaming for your attention. I like to think of solitude as a gift. Solitude in your car, on an early morning road trip with your favorite music, is a whole other thing than being alone in your car surrounded by ten thousand other cars, the traffic helicopter whirring, and listening to the reports of the stock market wavering on the brink of recession.

Practice going alone sometimes. Maybe not every time you exercise, but as part of your regimen of inconsistency. Join a new group, take a new class, without the support of a buddy you already know. You may feel like a shy nine-year-old starting at a new school, but you can do it. Without the history that your old friends and family bring to your attempts at athleticism, you can be liberated to try a new exercise persona. Don't let the fear of being on your own stop you from pursuing the dream.

THE LOWDOWN: MAKING THE WORDS REAL

Think of an off-the-wall activity you've always wanted to try. Climbing at the indoor gym? Speed skating? Extreme pogoing? Boxing? Tae kwon do? Now go find it. This is why Google was invented, so that you could find the most fun things to do in your neck of the woods. Maybe you have to expand the definition of your neck of the woods to include a slightly thicker neck, but there are a lot of activities. Now pick up the phone and call the people who can get you started. Then go by yourself. Make a point of going by yourself. If you like it, you can take a friend the next time. But being willing to try new stuff by yourself builds the adventurous spirit that all athletes, especially imperfect ones, need to have.

On a smaller scale, try getting out for a ten-minute walk by yourself. On your work break or right after you get home, whenever. This is totally related to the idea of being selfish. Don't accommodate anyone's schedule. Just go.

31

GO WITH FRIENDS

IF YOU WANT to go alone, go alone. But if you want to go with friends, hey, get the whole crowd together. Or alternate. Be inconsistent. Anyhow, if you want to turn your athletic endeavors into an extension of your social life, I'm all behind that. It's awesome. But you're going to have to figure out how to get those friends to sign up and train with you.

As much as I extol the joys of solitary exercising, the social aspects of fitness can be a big bonus, and if you can get people to come out and discover a new sport with you, it can deepen and strengthen your friendship in all kinds of wonderful ways. The people who helped shove me onto my current path to imperfect athleticism had no idea what a monster they were creating, but we had a lot of extra fun in doing running and triathlon events together. When I asked my old friend and triathlete buddy Russ what the sporty stuff added to our friendship, he answered, "Well, come on, now we share a whole other common language." I thought back on this and remembered the time when we both did the San Jose International Triathlon on an exceptionally windy morning. After the race, Russ and I were talking

157

about our strategy for cycling into the headwind, and I said to him, "Well, I got lucky and caught a legal draft behind a wide-body on a tricked-out softtail." Russ said, "I love that I know exactly what you mean by that."

When you get your old friends or your sister or brother-in-law to take up a new sporty endeavor with you, you can share the surprising discoveries that you might be too embarrassed to share with new acquaintances. Like all the body parts that can get chafed, numb, or sore when you first take up cycling and you haven't yet worked out the right combo of shorts, saddle, and antichafing technologies. Unless you're a gal like me, for whom the warning "too much information!" was invented, you may not want to talk about your coochie pains with the members of the cycling club you just joined two weeks ago.

You can research equipment and share training tips with your friends and family. You can share the burden of figuring out what you need, what the rules are, what the vocabulary means, whether you will need to upgrade your medical coverage, all the confusing stuff.

Or you can use your circle of friends to teach each other about compassion, determination, perseverance, the uses of planning versus the uses of letting things flow, and the excitement of shared victory even when some of you are much "better" at the sport than others. Those are all good things to do with your friends or family too.

Beth, the onetime gnarly kayaker, has a new approach to her fitness these days, and it totally includes the family:

> Throughout my years of running rivers, of cutting-edge expeditions, of first descents in exotic lands, I believed it was my right to selfishly devote myself to fitness. I did whatever it took to

stay out front, so that I could hold my own in those remote river canyons, so that the U.S. Women's Whitewater Team would continuously be on the podium at World Championships. What I didn't know was that the surge in self-esteem that comes from elite fitness would not last forever. With the hubris of youth, I believed that aging happens to others.

Three years after my daughter's birth, I can once again hold myself upright in a kayak thanks to Pilates and a lot of hard work. But instead of running waterfalls, I plan family adventures where everyone gets to be a hero. Family life is the richest thing there is, though I'd be lying if I said I didn't miss life out there on the edge.

You can work with your friends and family to make all your exercise-related activities more fun. Create competitions for the silliest slogans for your event or goal. "The Fabulous Fifteen-Minute-Mile Megalomaniac Munchkins Marching Merrily to May 15."

Here are a couple of things to keep in mind as you gather your friends together.

Not all your friends have the same goals as you. One person may just want to finish the event and not be last (though I personally think that coming in last is perfectly fine); another may want to do the event in a certain time or in his or her own particular . . . idiom. I once ran a 5k in Palm Springs with Indigo while Russ was doing a half marathon. Also, one of Indigo's priorities was to do the whole 5k while juggling three orange balls. Which she did, with only one drop per kilometer. And her juggling kept her closer to my running pace. Afterward, we both hung out and cheered on other runners until Russ came to the line. So think about ways you can all accommodate each other's athletic ambitions.

You are probably not all going to be at the same level of ability in your new sport. Even if none of you has ever played ice hockey before or even been on skates, some people are going to have better balance and pick up skills more quickly. It's just that way. Some people are less imperfect than others. If anyone in your group is going to be all mean-girly about it and flaunt her superiority, or conversely turn into a mopey buzzkill because she falls on her butt more often than the rest of you, this could mess up your dynamic. On the other hand, you may decide that these aren't the people you want around as you undertake things that are supposed to be fun.

If your friends are also your coworkers, think carefully about whether you want to get together with them in any sport where they could see you naked, like swimming or mud wrestling. And then abandon self-consciousness and do it anyway.

Decide if you want to focus your group energies on an athletic event for charity, as described in Chapter 7. A cause can inspire you to greater heights of teamwork and camaraderie, and it can help smooth over potential frictions around training schedules, ability levels, or willingness to go the extra mile. Besides, you can pool your energies to do your fund-raising.

Organize a group event around movement, rather than, say, sitting around and quaffing mojitos or beers. Evite is the best thing since sliced bread for getting family and friends together. Make it a group hike at a site with various options for people with varying levels of hiking ambition and endurance, and do a big-ass picnic afterward. Or create your own volleyball tournament, even if you have to buy a ball and a net and download the rules that you haven't thought about since grade school.

If it's your girlfriends, put together Ladies' Crazy Dance Night at a local club. If you're old like me, wait for 80s Night or

Disco Night, or clear out the furniture and make your own club. Have Dance Dance Revolution tournament, so you can hang with your peeps and get your move on at the same time. DDR is an awesome workout. Put your mat down, plug in your PlayStation (or your kids' PlayStation) and let 'er rip.

Or you could bribe your fifteen-year old to teach you how the kids are dancing these days. And if you're shocked, don't show it. It's just dancing. People used to think that the Charleston was obscene. Now it's quaint.

BE NONCOMPETITIVE

I AM A somewhat competitive person. I can't usually beat my husband Tim at Scrabble, but I still try, and my glee when I do pull out a win verges on the unseemly. Put a basketball in my hands, and no matter how long it has been since I last flaunted my crossover dribble, I'll still believe that I can take you to the hoop, even if I have to run you over to do it. I'll bump you with my behind, knock you off balance, and bank a gentle hook shot off the backboard.

So how is it that I am espousing noncompetitiveness? Is this not akin to Bubba the barbecue chef exhorting the public to convert to a vegan diet? Maybe. "Do as I say, not as I do" has become my mantra as an imperfect fitness guru. I'm not saying that competitiveness is bad. Properly directed and channeled, competitiveness can be a force for fun. But that's a different subject. This chapter is about not being competitive, about not wanting to kick ass, about being Ferdinand the Bull and choosing to smell the flowers in the middle of the field rather than butt heads with the macho bulls.

Mainstream American culture values competitiveness: better, stronger, faster, higher achieving. Nice guys finish last. Winning isn't everything, it's the only thing. No disrespect to Vince Lombardi, but clearly winning isn't the only thing. If it were, you wouldn't have 40,000 people signed up to run the Chicago Marathon. At least 38,750 of those people know they have no chance to win, and their Chicago Marathon experience will not be one whit less valuable for all that. Obviously winning isn't even a consideration for most of these people. Even finishing in the top ten or twenty in their age-groups is not a consideration. The main consideration is the experience.

If you're not worried about how you're going to do relative to the person next to you, you can concentrate on learning what you're doing and enjoying it. Triathlon writer Amy White, in a charming article on "lunatics" of the sport, lauds obscure Italian triathlete Gino Petri, who once did three laps of a bike course that he was supposed to only do twice, just because he thought the scenery was pretty. This was not a guy who let competitiveness get in the way of having a good time.

Competitiveness as an ingrained trait makes you afraid to try things you might not necessarily be good at. I, for example, have certain athletic talents. These include strength, hand-eye coordination, considerable agility for a big girl, and a willingness to be physically aggressive. My talents came in handy playing basketball, softball, and rugby. I've never shown any talent for speed as a runner, I have no background in competitive swimming, and my build makes it unlikely that I will ever be much of a cyclist, especially when it comes to going uphill. So if I had gone into the sport of triathlon with the intent of being competitive, I would've been unhappy right away.

Sure, I could concentrate on competing against myself. And in fact I have done so. I savored my improving times, my increased efficiency, my gradual ascent up the ranks of my age-group, and especially in the ranks of the Athena class (triathlon-speak for big girl). But when I started getting fatter and slower, I had to find different things to enjoy about training and racing.

In this process, I had to take lessons from Indigo, the only person I know who has studied kickboxing for years and has no desire to get in the ring for a bout, let alone kick somebody's ass and break his kneecaps. "I had never had anyone try to hit me in my life. I had no concept of self-defense and couldn't imagine intentionally trying to hurt someone else," she said. Indigo enjoys learning the skills, training with serious fighters, kicking the heavy bag until her shins turn blue. She ran a 5k race with me at a pace that was barely more than a jog for her, just to keep me company. She did a triathlon in Newport Beach with me and her friend Dorli, and she sang, "I want to ride my bicycle, I want to ride my bike" throughout the entire bike ride. This is a woman who seriously does not care where her name ends up on the results list.

I think it's partly because Indigo is so unconcerned about competing that she has tried so many sports and activities and had so much fun doing them. She has climbed rock faces in Joshua Tree, sea kayaked along the California coast, rafted rivers in Russia, ridden her bike solo across the United States, learned salsa dancing, and developed such a powerful roundhouse kick that she has knocked the heavy bag clear off its hook. Here's how Indigo describes her experience as a kickboxer:

Three years ago I started cardio kickboxing classes, learning the basics of jabs and hooks at lunchtime classes with athletic house-wives and retired ladies from the neighborhood. I had never seen

a boxing match and knew nothing about Muay Thai kickboxing. My coaches were young guys who taught cardio classes and
worked other jobs to support themselves while they trained for
their next big fight. As I listened to their stories about strategic
attacks and defensive moves, I became intrigued. I started at-
tending local fights to support my coaches. My workouts shifted
from strictly cardio to more fight-specific techniques and I
started training one-on-one with other people like me.

For the most part I forget that I don't belong there—a middle-
aged white woman strolling into the sacred training room reserved primarily for the pros. Even though I wear the shorts and
the gloves of a Muay Thai kickboxer, I am not one of them. I am
old enough to be most of these guys' mother. I have no tattoos; I
have never been in a street fight. I am not like them, but I think
they have gotten used to me being here. I admit, I do fantasize
about someday stepping into the ring for a real bout. But for now,
I sweat, I learn, and I cheer them on as best as I can—and try to
get used to the otherworldly, can't-believe-this-is-happening-to-
me feeling I get every time I climb into the ring.

Every once in a while my coach's coach will invite me to put
my gear on and climb into the ring with real fighters. For a few
minutes, I try and hit them as hard and fast as I can, and they are
not allowed to hit back, only block. Some of the fighters will
laugh and smile behind their head gear; they know I will do
them no harm and the quickness of their response is thrilling.
They know what I will try before I do, and I am no threat to
them. Others switch into their "fight face." Eyes that dance with
mischief outside of the ring now stare back at me with a fierce
intensity that makes me want to run. For the most part, I am
a mosquito swarming around their ears. Sometimes I can land a
punch, which always brings me up short with surprise. And

when I manage to sneak one in, the fighters usually respond with a smile and nod of approval. They did teach me after all.

This is the great thing: Indigo has studied the psychology of fighting in considerable depth, but she has no urge to get in the ring in a real fight. And I think that's why she has been able to learn so much. Me, I'd be so eager to get in the ring and crush someone that I'd probably miss out on all the nuances that Indi has picked up.

So if you're like me and you feel your competitive juices starting to simmer in a group of your peers, or you're hesitating to do something new because you think you might not be good at it, follow the example of Indigo or Gino. Sing a song instead of working too hard. Ride an extra lap so you come in last. Nobody's paying you to do this stuff. It's child's play.

THE LOWDOWN: MAKING THE WORDS REAL

How can you modulate your competitive instincts or conditioning so that you have more fun and less angst? A few ideas.

Run with someone slower than you. Let her set the pace.

If you're already participating in timed events, do one without your watch. Focus on the scenery. Count the species of birds you see, or models of cars or state license plates. For really advanced noncompetitiveness, don't look up your results on the web later.

Try something you know you're not good at, either because you're a raw beginner or you've tried it before and your efforts were laughable. Then laugh at your efforts. I use triathlon for this purpose, but I can always fall back on bowling if I find myself getting too chippy.

Organize a wrong-handed bocce tournament: everyone has to throw with the opposite hand.

33

DON'T MAKE THE DONUT THE REWARD

I WAS ABOUT four miles into a 10k race one rainy April morning, trotting through the streets of San Jose, and I mean it was really, seriously, mega-raining. Soaked to the skin in seconds (fortunately I was not wearing cotton clothing), sloshing through ankle-deep puddles in a crowd of thousands of runners, I was having a perfectly lovely time. The rain was keeping me cool; I had paced myself just as I had planned; my fellow runners were a cheerful bunch, and I wasn't suffering at all. We were proceeding at a moderate pace through residential neighborhoods, and as we rounded one corner, a woman stood on the sidewalk cheering us on with the most inspiring cheer she could think of: "Think of the huge breakfast you can eat after this!"

I appreciated her getting out there with her umbrella and supporting the runners, but her exhortation was a little off base. I hadn't given much thought to my postrace breakfast. I suppose I was going to eat a little more than I normally would on a Sunday morning, but I wasn't out there running 6.2 miles so that I could have a guilt-free chowfest of pancakes, bacon, eggs, and hash browns. Believe it or not, I was out there running just because I wanted to.

The nice umbrella woman's assumption about why we exercise is pervasive among exercisers and nonexercisers alike. Exercise, in this philosophy, is something you do in order to earn food rewards (30 minutes on the Stairmaster equals one mocha, except it doesn't) or punish yourself for food sins (one mocha equals 30 minutes on the treadmill, except it doesn't). You think about your workout in terms of guilt and redemption, sin and expatiation. It's puritanical, it devalues exercise, and it makes me mad (though of course that doesn't stop me from engaging in it myself). Furthermore, Sally Edwards points out that the simple equation of calories in, calories out doesn't even work when it comes to regular exercise. Sally has a huge list of books, a training business, and a massive athletic resume, so she should know. The thing is that as we do a certain exercise over a period of weeks or months, our bodies become more efficient at that exercise and begin to burn fewer calories. So your 30 minutes on the treadmill at intensity level 6 burns fewer calories in the twelfth week of your exercise adventure than it did in the first week. So don't even think about that equation.

When you couple your exercise to your right to eat certain foods or use the exercise to atone for eating the food, it adds a layer of psychological complication to what should be a much simpler motivation. You take exercise from its own realm and put it into the murkier territory of all the things you feel guilty about. Your weight, your heart, your cholesterol, the number of vegetables you do or don't eat, the amount of time you spend at work or don't spend at work—all the horrid obligations and vague worries of modern life. You're constantly working out little equations of what you have to do in order to work off what you ate or what you're planning to eat.

And, as I mentioned above, most of us are extremely bad at estimating the relative values of those equations. Take the example above. Using a couple of Web calculators (and measuring your calories burned is only a game of estimating unless you get into some fancy high-tech testing), I figured that a 160-pound person would burn about 230 calories during a 30-minute session on a stair-stepping machine. That same stair-stepping person, having showered and changed, or alternatively just toweled off and jumped in the car, might then reward herself with a grande mocha at Starbucks and, thinking always in terms of virtue, order it without whipped cream. That would be 300 calories there. Add a virtuous-sounding low-fat blueberry muffin, and that's another 340 calories. So now you're 410 calories in the red, and you wonder why you work out and work out and can't lose weight. That's why. If like me, you weigh 250 pounds, you might burn 350 to 380 calories on the stair torturer, but you'd still end up almost 300 calories in the hole with your mocha/muffin combo. And thirty minutes on the stair machine is a bear. It's hard work, and it seems like you should get at least a nice little bevy and a pastry out of it. But no, you don't.

So my sense is that if you're always working out with an eye to your caloric allowance, you're going to be sadly disappointed. And being sadly disappointed is not a recipe for fun.

I don't want to say that a really long, tough workout or event doesn't merit the occasional super burrito, pizza fest, or fried breakfast extravaganza. We're all only human, and proudly imperfect in our humanity. I can recall any number of occasions on which I ate more than any nutritionist would advise after a triathlon or a four-hour bike ride. But as a rule, you have to work your body vigorously for several hours at a stretch before that level of indulgence applies. And my real point is not to base your motivation for your regular exercise on the food involved. Food is a separate issue, or maybe a bunch of separate issues.

Yes, you need sugar to fuel your workout, but your body can make it out of lots of different substances. Move for the sake of movement, not for a donut.

THE LOWDOWN: MAKING THE WORDS REAL

Movement is its own reward, in my book. And this is my book, as it happens. During your workout focus on the following factors:

Are you enjoying your movement?
Are you challenging yourself to the degree you want?
Are you moving as easily and efficiently as you can under the circumstances?
Are you chafing? (If so, see Chapter 22.)

And not necessarily in that order. After your workout, try and figure out exactly what your body is hungry for. It may not be hungry for anything right away. Or it may want a bit of fruit or some graham crackers. And plenty of water. You may or may not want a big meal later on. Just think about what you really want, and why.

BE AN ACTIVEWEAR ACTIVIST

YOUR CHRONIC SENSE of imperfection does not necessarily stem from the sheer volume of your bod. Sadly, most of us, regardless of size, can feel put upon by athletic clothing. Especially with all those designer sweatsuits (in which you probably should not sweat) in sizes tiny, extra tiny, and supremely wee.

Throughout my career as an imperfect athlete I have been plagued by the mind-set and marketing decisions of the manufacturers of athletic apparel. This is tough for all of us, but for any woman larger than a size 14 or so, the options for clothing yourself for your chosen sport in a way that is simultaneously functional, comfortable, and cute are nearly nonexistent. Even if you take cute out of the equation, which I am usually willing to do, the choices are still limited. Few companies recognize that larger women are not universally immobile, bolted to the couch with an automatic bonbon feeder set to force a tasty tidbit down their throats at three-minute intervals.

Let us give our props to these companies, the ones who make quality fitness wear for women of quantity and are happy to advertise that fact. Danskin. Terry. Junonia. Moving Comfort, Shebeest, REI. Big ol' "woo-hoo" to you. Props. Word. Champion makes a few items. There's also SportHill, Pizzazz, and A Big Attitude. SportHill features the most technical fabrics, while the Pizzazz and ABA folks are heavier on cotton, about which, as you know, I am dubious. At least as far as exercise wear. I'm delighted that more companies are getting hip to the idea of a large new market even as I write, but we large athletes need more.

Target makes Target-quality fitness wear in plus sizes. You can do "regular" workouts in their stuff but not a three-hour marathon training run. No offense to Target, but that's not their market. Target's for the basics. When you want something that'll do fine and you don't have to worry about wrecking it, you go to Target. (This is why so much of my work apparel budget goes to Target.)

What bugs me is walking into a store that is supposedly dedicated to helping people become more fit and finding that the largest women's top in the whole place would not be particularly baggy on my mom, who's 5'1" and weighs 124 pounds. Actually, a lot of times the women's size XL tops wouldn't be all that baggy on my cat, who's twenty-eight inches long from nose to tail and weighs about fourteen pounds.

I have taken to polite activewear activism, especially in the sports specialty stores that capture my $112 for fresh running shoes three to four times a year. I stroll up to the counter or to the wandering salesperson and say sweetly, "Excuse me, where are your plus size women's clothes?" Almost inevitably the salesperson will look embarrassed (especially if he's a boy) and say, "I'm sorry, we don't have any." Sometimes, if I'm feeling particularly activistic, I'll hold a teeny-weeny size XL top next to my size 44DDD torso and say, "Well, now, tell me honestly, how is a woman who's my size supposed to train in this? *This* is an extra large? Take a look at this body, honey. *That* is an extra large. And I'm a triathlete, not a couch potato, okay?"

Usually by this point the salesperson is squirming and looking desperately for someone else to assist. And because I'm not actually a mean person, I usually let him or her off the hook with a small lecture about how not every woman who does active stuff is built to fit into this little item (as I hold up the tiny workout top again), and as a regular consumer of athletic gear, I would be pleased to find something in the women's section that I could wear. Sometimes, if I'm feeling particularly activist, I ask to talk to the manager. Then I walk off, head held high, to buy another men's size XL or XXL running shirt.

Rebecca from Washington, who is a lot smaller than I am, shares my frustrations on this score:

It has not been easy to be a big, strong athletic woman. Sports clothing manufacturers do not believe larger-busted women are supposed to play sports. Thank goodness for the Internet! And who in the hell ever invented the uni-boob style sports bra? Obviously no one with larger than an A cup! You know, the flatten-your-breasts-into-one-wide-pancake-style sports bra, the kind that looks absolutely ridiculous on breasts larger than a small plum? And just try to find a swimsuit for lap swimming that will adequately cover large shoulders and breasts but doesn't sag on small hips and a smaller butt. Find volleyball or running shoes for DDDD wide feet with really high insteps? Just try to find a wetsuit on the rack if you're a larger and/or odd-shaped woman. And don't even get me started on running or cycling clothes.

I have e-mailed some large companies (which will remain nameless for now), asking them why they have blatantly failed to address the abundant market for fitness wear for millions of American and international nonstick-figures. I invariably receive an automated response saying something like, "Thank-you for your ~~ridiculous~~ question. International Sweatshop, Inc., highly values your opinion and a customer service representative will contact you shortly with a personalized response to your ~~deluded~~ request." I can almost hear the laughter coming over the e-mail connection.

You have a supremely practical need for clothes that work for you when you exercise. Your exercise clothes are tools, and you need functional tools. And if there are more of us out there demanding the tools we need, maybe we'll actually get them.

Obviously the issue of big girls getting access to the same variety and quality of clothes that skinny girls have is beyond the scope of this book. There are social, political, economic, and public health aspects to the question, and they can all be debated till the cows come home (but those cows will not be wearing teeny-weeny sports tops). Why do clothing manufacturers, media moguls, and race organizers

- Believe we should all conform to a particular body type?
- Tell us that the only way to get to that body type is through exercise?
- Refuse to make us clothes that we can wear to exercise in?

So ask for the clothes you want, and keep asking until you get them. Until we get them.

REBEL AGAINST NUMBERS

WE ARE TYRANNIZED by numbers. From the creeping deductions in our paychecks to the inexorable march of the dashboard clock, from the ridiculous oversimplification of the body mass index to the plummeting definition of what constitutes healthy blood pressure, numbers run our lives. You are in thrall to your bathroom scale, your (never sufficient) IRA contributions, the value of your house, the interest rate on your favorite credit card, your pants size, your grade point average, the miles you've driven since your last oil change.

This chapter is about not letting numbers rule your life as an imperfect athlete. The most critical numbers to ignore are your age, your weight, and any indicators of your performance in your chosen sport. Obviously you should get your doctor to check you out before indulging in strenuous physical effort so you don't get blindsided by a sneaky little heart condition or what not, but your doctor will probably say it's okay. In the words of fat chick aerobics instructor Jeanette de Patie, "I'm guessing he actually started jumping up and down when you asked him saying, *yes yes yes, so let's stop procrastinating and start right now!*"

Generally speaking, the older and/or fatter you are, the more cautiously you should approach your sport. Age predisposes most people to injuries. We lose flexibility, and recovering from hard effort takes longer. Weight puts strain on your joints and your cardiopulmonary system, relative to someone with the same fitness level and less body weight. These things are generally true. But you can still do the things you want to do. As my husband is fond of pointing out, statistics are meaningless at the individual level. Just because some vanishingly small percentage of octogenarians are first-time triathletes, that doesn't mean you can't do your first triathlon at the age of eighty-one.

I had the honor of being present at just such a debut at the Abitaman, a small but devastatingly beautiful race in Navarre Beach, Florida. The final finisher came in at a stately shuffle quite a while after most competitors were enjoying jambalaya on the restaurant deck, but the race announcer gathered us together to give her a huge ovation. Then the announcer asked eighty-one-year-old Margaret what the hardest part of the race had been. "The bicycle seat," she replied. So don't tell me you can't do a triathlon just because you're over eighty. Or over three hundred pounds for that matter, because I've seen that happen plenty of times too.

For Margaret, her finishing time was hardly the point of the exercise. If she did another triathlon later on (and I do hope she did because she seemed to be enjoying herself), she might have spared a thought for whether she was faster or slower her second time out than her first. Or not. Either way, the glory of her successful participation, of being outside on a beautiful

April morning on a beach so white it looked like cane sugar, was hardly diminished by her speed or lack of same.

I'm not denigrating the human urge to compete (see Chapter 32), and I'm not saying you shouldn't track your performances, compare your average pace per mile from one race to another, even compare your placing within your age-group or how you did against that gal from Fair Oaks who always seems to be two minutes ahead of you. Those things are all fine and dandy, as long as they don't keep you from enjoying the activity itself. If you find that you're not enjoying the activity because the numbers aren't right, then for Pete's sake quit watching the numbers. Just cut it out.

The numbers are all a game, and I urge you to treat them as such (assuming you pay attention to them at all). If you start obsessing about your performance numbers, go back and review Chapters 3–5. You're not getting evaluated on this stuff; your paycheck, fortunately, doesn't depend on it, and neither should your self-esteem.

Please. Don't decide to do a marathon (or anything else) because of the numbers on the scale, or on the clock, or on your birth certificate. Do it for its own sake, because it's a gratifying and engrossing thing to do. Unshackle yourself from the rule of numbers, from measurements, from timing, from poundage, from performance.

36

REGARD ALARMIST HEALTH NEWS WITH SKEPTICISM

TRANS FATS, GOOD cholesterol, bad cholesterol. Salt is bad for you, dark chocolate is good for you. Oh, wait, salt is probably not so bad, but bread is bad. No, bread is okay. Good fats, bad fats, good carbs, bad carbs. Eat more fatty fish; no, wait, watch out for the fatty fish. It might have mercury residue in it. Drinking moderate amounts of alcohol (one or two drinks per day) can have beneficial effects for heart health (two years ago). "Drinking alcohol at moderate levels—two or more drinks per day—appears to be a risk factor for abdominal aortic aneurysm in men, researchers found" (today). Abdominal aortic aneurysm kills the heck out of you in just a few minutes, as your aorta ruptures and your heart pumps gouts of blood straight into your insides. So watch that Bud Light! Hormone replacement seemed to be the best thing since sliced bread (which is now okay as long as it's whole grain) for menopausal women, right up until it caused breast cancer, heart attacks, or strokes.

It doesn't take Dr. House to see where I'm going here. We are bombarded by alarmist health news on a daily basis. If you want, you can probably find at least three different things to worry about in each day's media offerings. And yesterday's medical certainty can be today's ill-founded belief. Call it progress; call it the march of science. Definitely call it an out-of-control media machine that values eyeballs (and eardrums) far more than an in-depth analysis of the relative risks and benefits, let alone the relative degree of certainty of the scary thing du jour. People get exposed to new medical information or misinformation, and they start to obsess about it. And it's not just the "real news" that's in play here. There's a medical doctor who runs a blog with great reviews of every episode of *House*, and he says that he's had at least three patients convinced they had the disease of the week from the series.

We don't really know what's going to get us in the end. So in my view, basing your exercise or dietary habits on the constantly changing news of the day is irrational and creates a whole heap of unnecessary stress in your life.

Exercise because it's fun and it's good for you in general. Eat for the same reasons. I have certain principles which, when I follow them, make me feel I'm nourishing my body and my psyche. I'll share them, though I hope you'll develop your own.

Eat foods that Thomas Jefferson would recognize, things such as rice, turnips, beans, milk, cheese, eggs, oats, cabbage, walnuts, spinach, strawberries, and so on. Bacon-cheddar flavored Cheetos, Double Stuf Oreos, Pringles, and Fruity Pebbles were not in Jefferson's pantry. Bacon cheeseburgers? Well, why not?

Jefferson would have known about ground beef, bacon, cheese, and bread rolls, even if he didn't combine them in the way we know and love. Why Thomas Jefferson? I think Michael Pollan wrote about him in one of his really cool books about plants and food. Jefferson was a farmer and enthusiastic gardener who introduced exotic foods and dishes (including ice cream; what a great, great man) from Europe to the kitchens at Monticello and the White House. I just think of him as a dude who liked food and liked to be healthy, a handy measuring stick for whether something is "real food" or not.

Eat vegetarian frequently. Rice and beans are good. They taste good and they fuel you up and you can do lots of different things with them. Beans have tons of fiber, plenty of protein, a bundle of carbs for energy, trace minerals, and even folate, which may help prevent heart disease (or not, depending on the medical news of the week). Cook them well, add Beano if you have trouble with gas, and enjoy. Rice, and by that I mean brown rice, has essential fatty acids, manganese, selenium, magnesium, and all kinds of good stuff. I always feel clean when I eat a bunch of brown rice and vegetables. Even tofu, maligned by carnivores everywhere, can be tasty with a good marinade and a quick grilling, and it's full of protein and iron.

Eating spreads instead of butter or olive oil just ain't worth it. Neither is nonfat salad dressing, low-fat cheese, or nonfat milk. I didn't get to be fat using 1 percent milk on my cereal. Even spreads without "hydrogenated this" or "trans-fatty that" are still foods processed to within an inch of their lives. Would Jefferson eat them? I don't think so. But real butter and good olive oil are wonderful even in small amounts. I like them in large amounts too, but that's my cross to bear. Eating a little "real" fat gives you a lot more satisfaction because fat is what nature puts in food to make it taste good. Seriously, many chemical compounds that we perceive as "yummy" are transported only by fat. No fat, no flavor.

And don't even get me started on fat-free salad dressings. Look at what's in those things—modified food starch, guar gum, carrageenan—all things to thicken the dressing and make it feel like something in your mouth. Tim refers to these dressings as "thick water." But I think of them as "thick water with all kinds of weird crap in it." Try buttermilk and spices—salt, pepper, garlic, onion, and parsley. Or pour a teaspoon of really great olive oil over your salad, shake a tiny bit of balsamic vinegar on it, and toss it with salt and pepper. So-o-o good.

Only eat really high-quality chocolate. It tastes amazing and it's the only kind of chocolate I can eat in small quantities without immediately wanting more.

Have one drink. Not a six-pack or a bottle.

Pay attention to the things you crave. Author and fitness mega-guru Sally Edwards believes that if you crave a certain food, it's probably not that good for your personal metabolism. When you experience cravings, you might want to think about how to balance what you eat so that you have fewer of them.

Eat when hungry; stop when full. This is a hard principle to adhere to, and it's the one that marketing and advertising work hardest to subvert. It's also the ultimate healthy eating advice. Practice paying attention to what hunger feels like, and what fullness means to your body. Learn to recognize the two.

My guess is that if you follow these broad guidelines most of the time, then that's going to mitigate a lot of the risks that may be lurking in your food. You can seek after perfect health to a greater degree, of course. You can frequent farmers markets and buy organic produce, dairy, eggs, meat. You can grow your own veggies. You can eschew whole categories of food (meat, dairy, whatever). But I don't think you have to. If your forays into the processed food mazes of Burger King and Cheez-Its are occasional rather than habitual, if you have a lot of whole grains, legumes, vegetables, and fruits in your pantry (and you actually eat them), and you sometimes eat reasonable quantities of fun rich things like chocolate and stinky French cheeses and USDA prime beef, then you're probably in decent shape, risk-wise. If, on top of these generally healthy dietary practices, you also move your body regularly, get your sleep, drink your water, and don't do really silly things like smoke or take street drugs, then quit worrying and live.

SECTION V

SEVEN ADVANCED WORKOUTS FOR YOUR MIND

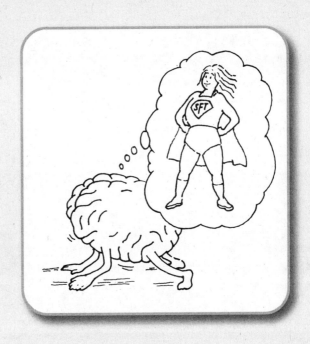

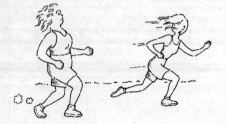

STUDY YOUR BODY
Nuts and Bolts

YOUR BODY IS way cool. Regardless of what you think about its superficial features—hair color, level of sports accomplishment, or how it looks in a slinky evening gown—your body is fabulously, infinitely cool. The mechanics of your musculature, the flexibility of your fascia, the tensile strength of your tendons, the miracle of your mitochondria. The simple act of getting up off the couch involves, among other things, hundreds of moving parts, the firing of thousands of neurons, the coordination of your proprioceptors that help your brain position your body in space, the transformation of a minute amount of blood glucose into fuel for the operation.

Back in the early 1990s, I used to get bodywork (they never call it massage) from a certified Rolfer. He manipulated my muscles and soft tissues so that my whole body lines up straight and true, as it did when I was a kid. He would explain to me which muscles he was tormenting and what they were for. I learned about the iliopsoas, the gluteus minimus, the quadratus lumborum and the always-good-for-a-scream-of-agony inter-costals (these connect your ribs one to another; you would not believe how tight they get just from everyday office life). There are also fascia, which bundle muscles together in tight little packages. Sometimes those packages get wrapped too tightly, and that can make things hurt.

At the time I was getting Rolfed, I was working actively on my fitness: running, riding my bike, even playing some one-on-one hoops now and then, using my always sturdy rear to back down in the low post. So I was able to observe the effects of each session of bodywork out in the field. I was able to feel when my feet felt balanced under my torso, when my shoulders were level instead of crooked, when my hips moved freely instead of feeling stiff and constricted. And those things felt good.

However, Rolfing did not prevent pains and strains from re-curring, and so my knowledge of muscles, bones, ligaments, fas-cia, and tendons was propelled forward by my various injuries. I learned that there are a lot of muscles that enable your hips to flex (raise your knee toward your torso) when I strained a bunch of them during an aerobics class. There is the mighty il-iopsoas, the sartorius, the pectineus, and the tensor fasciae latae, or "the thing that tenses the fascia of the side." I learned about my gastrocnemius and my soleus when I had Achilles tendonitis after a long backpacking trip. My trusty chiropractor and physical therapist, Petra Eggert, has taught me about every-thing from my trapezius to my erector spinae ("the thing that holds your spine upright") over the ten-plus years I've been having her fix my ongoing ills. "Understanding the functions of your muscles can help you prevent injuries," she agrees. "But you do have to do the work to strengthen and stretch the mus-cles; otherwise knowing about them won't do you any good."

You might think that all the injuries and tweaks I've endured would make me (1) sick and tired of learning about muscles and tendons and (2) sensible enough to just sit on the couch and watch other people exert themselves through the magic of television. But just the opposite has happened. The more I learn about how the different muscle groups work together, the more fascinated I am by the strength, complexity, and adaptability of the body. And the process of being injured and then healing has given me a profound appreciation of the body's ability to renew itself, as well as a determination to stretch and strengthen the right things in the right way so that I don't get hurt again. This determination usually lasts right up to the point where nothing hurts, at which point I abandon the dull routines of stretching and strengthening in favor of stuff I think is more fun. Then I get hurt again. There are some lessons you have to learn over and over before you actually internalize them. When I am hurting, I find it pleasing and comforting to know what hurts and why.

What's even cooler, though, is to understand what gets stronger as you exercise, and how you can keep getting stronger and gaining endurance by taking care of those muscles and tendons. Most of us don't apply anywhere near the same diligence to our bodily maintenance as we do to our cars, and we end up with the biomechanical equivalent of cracked belts, worn-out shocks, clogged fuel lines, and weakened axles. But with a little study of your owner's manual, you can get better performance for longer.

THE LOWDOWN: MAKING THE WORDS REAL

If you want to learn about the workings of your bod, do it in an orderly way. Get a book out of the library or buy *The Anatomy Coloring Book* (seriously!) and try coloring your own quadratus lumborum. Or check out some of the diagrams and interactive tutorials on the web; those med schools have great stuff. I bought the American Council on Exercise study guide to becoming a personal trainer, which covers exercise physiology as well as muscle group anatomy. Then you can start to study the crazy mad-scientist bubbling test tube that makes your cells work: your own body. Just open a cover and let 'er rip. Try it on a schedule:

Weeks 1–2: Major muscles of the legs: calf, hamstrings, quadriceps, sartorius, and so forth.

Weeks 3–4: Major muscles of the torso. What keeps your middle from slumping over like a bean bag?

Weeks 5–6: Upper body: arms, shoulders (including the treacherous rotator cuff), neck.

Weeks 7–8: How the interaction of legs and torso combine to make you powerful. In other words, the function of muscles of "the core." Learn why straight up stomach crunches are of limited value in the real world.

Weeks 9–10: Hands and feet. Feet are crucial to most athletic endeavors. Learn about how they work and why they are easily injured. If you spend forty hours a week at the computer keyboard, read up about how to keep your hands from getting hurt so they don't keep you from swinging a bat or riding a bike.

I'm not saying this has to be as grueling as a college class in anatomy and physiology. Just google "major muscles of the leg" when you have five minutes of down time. Don't worry too much about the minute details, like memorizing the names of every metatarsal bone or tiny tendon of the hand. Focus on the movers and shakers.

REVEL IN THE
JOYS OF DATA

THERE IS NO reason you can't be an athlete and a geek too. I think the two modes go well together. As you work to transform your cardiovascular capacity, core strength, flexibility, power, and balance, you are a laboratory of one. You are a walking, running, lifting, jumping science experiment, as well as a barely contained wild animal. You *are* applied biomechanics, biochemistry, and psychology. You may also be an experiment in sociology (as you work to change social norms by being a shame-free athlete), economics (if you get fired from your job for just saying no to extra work), and existential philosophy (you are what you actually do, not what you say you want to do).

There are many ways to gather and analyze data about your moving body. The simplest way, and the one on which many others are based, is to keep track of how you move, when you move, for how long, and how you feel when you do it. There are lots of online sites that will help you track your workout. Some are free; other are free initially and then want you to upgrade to a desktop software that you pay for, with the incentive of additional features. See the sidebar below for details. Just google "online workout journal" or "online exercise log" and poke around a bit. I'm not going to recommend any specific ones, since different setups work better for different people. There are also software packages you can buy for your home computer; or you can keep a spreadsheet. Or you can open up a spiral notebook and record your exercise sessions by hand.

I recommend electronic data keeping just because it helps you analyze trends. They may not emerge over a couple of weeks or even a couple of months, but as you build up a history of exercise sessions, you will start to see things happening. You may be able to run for forty-five minutes instead of twenty. You may feel better when you do it, or go at a faster pace. You may be able to complete all the heavy-bag kick sets after months of trying, or swim your 100s in 1:48, down from 2:12 six months ago. But if you don't record this, you won't truly appreciate the magnitude of your achievements.

How, you may ask, is this kind of geekery consistent with an ethos of fun? Glad you asked. Knowing stuff about yourself (always the most fascinating topic of all) is fun. It's interesting to see your abilities improve over time. If you take part in competitions, even just for the heck of it, it's cool to see how varying levels of preparation affect your performance.

Here's a sample of my spreadsheet-based training log. I've been using a system for triathletes developed by triathlon pioneer, inventor, writer, and uber-sports geek Dan Empfield, which allocates points to certain activities to balance your workload among swimming, cycling, running, and strength/core training. You get one point for every hundred yards you swim, one for every mile you ride, and four for every mile you

May	Swim mins.	Swim yds.	Bike mins.	Bike miles	Run mins.	Run miles	Core/Strength	POINTS	Weekly totals
1	36	1100					20	13	
2				13	40	2.3		9.2	
3			60				20	15	
4	40	1200	60	12	30	2		12	81.6
5					50	3.1		20	
6								12.4	
7								0	
8				14	40	2.4	10	9.6	
9			60		50	3.1		15	
10	40	1250	50	12			10	24.9	
11								13	96.9
12			90	20	60	3.6		14.4	
13	28	1000						20	
14							20	10	
15			60	12	30	2		10	
16								12	
17					30	2	20	10	
18	30	1100						11	62.2
19				0				0	
20			0		40	2.3		9.2	

run. I also wanted to see how many minutes I was putting into each session. Dan's got this chart online along with an explanation at www.slowtwitch.com/Training/Aerobic_points_system _15.html. ("Slow twitch" refers to the kinds of muscle fibers that endurance athletes tend to have more of. Athletes who excel at moving quickly in short bursts have more "fast twitch" muscles.)

This table helps me track my overall effort level over the course of the week. If I'm putting in 60 points worth of effort one week and 140 the next, that's an issue. It also helps me to schedule in recovery weeks every four weeks or so.

Recovery weeks involve shorter, less intense workouts that help consolidate the fitness gains of the preceding, more demanding weeks. The recovery week is an essential part of going slow and of taking two steps forward, one step back (see Chapters 3 and 16). If you use a table, you can see what your exercise workload has been week to week, and see when you need to schedule yourself a nice little break. So every four to six weeks, take your point value down by about half. It may seem wrong, but it's right.

If the table above sends you into a fit of anxiety or brings out a full-body rash, then you know what? Relax. Don't worry about it. Data collection and analysis are not mandatory for shaping up for or for being an athlete. To be an athlete, you have to sweat, but you don't have to geek out.

If, on the other hand, the table above sends you into a paroxysm of delight and fills you with an urge to create a much better, more detailed spreadsheet with running monthly totals, average calories burned per session, and data on temperature and relative humidity for each workout, including those conducted indoors, then I say to you, Dude. You are far, far crazier than I am.

There are, for better or worse, a number of handy gadgets that will help you burrow deeply into the world of sports data while simultaneously slimming unsightly bulges from your bank account. Paramount among these is the heart rate monitor (HRM), which, as the name suggests, monitors how many times your heart is beating per minute. The most common models combine a chest strap with a wrist watch or bike-mounted readout. The chest strap, besides adding a hint of kink to your workout ensemble, senses the pa-dump, pa-dump, pa-dump of your heartbeat and transmits that signal automagically to the little bitty computer in your watch, where a squad of gnomes transform the signal into a number you can read and perform a bunch of other complicated calculations to boot. Normal resting pulses range from forty beats per minute for Lance Armstrong to around eighty-five for sedentary computer jockeys amped to the eyeballs on Monster or Rock Star.

You don't need a personal trainer to do heart-rate based training. Sally Edwards, who among many other things is the "head heart" at HeartZones, Inc., has written a whole slew of books on the subject, which are practical, based on solid research, humane, and demystifying. Perfect for the entry level imperfect athlete. Sally points out, "The most important muscle in the body is the heart. The heart rate monitor helps you to get connected to your heart in a whole different way, both thinking about it and making an emotional connection to your body by feeling better about yourself." Sally claims that the most important thing is not to be looking at the number on the readout, but to be thinking about how you're "providing your heart with a language in which it can speak to you." Whether the number of beats per minute is going up, going down, or holding steady, your heart is telling you something about what it's experiencing. "It could be about the food you've been eating, your stress level, your hydration, overtraining. All of these affect your heart rate."

Strap on your chest transmitter, hit the start button on your wrist, and set off down the road, or along the treadmill, or up the trail, at whatever pace seems reasonable to you. Watch your heart rate go up as you exert yourself and go down as you ease off. This is entertaining, but the utility, not to mention statistical excitement, comes when you start looking at different zones of effort. The idea is that in exercising aerobically, different kinds of things are happening physiologically in the different zones. Some of these things have to do with glucose metabolism (see Chapter 21), others with the buildup of lactic acid, a by-product of glucose metabolism, in your bloodstream. By training strategically in these zones, you can boost your performance quite rapidly. My experience is that this really is true. The two seasons I trained with a coach (the ubiquitous and exemplary Coach Lisa Engles) using my HRM in this system were the two most amazing athletic years of my life—so far. Buy Sally Edwards's books and learn to train with your heart and your head.

So dive into data. Stretch your mind. Learn something. Apply your knowledge. Knowledge is power.

THE LOWDOWN: MAKING THE WORDS REAL

Plug in, tune in, turn on. There are several heart rate monitors on the market. Polar offers a variety of models ranging from supersimple (displays heart rate) to more complicated than I can get a handle on (predicts your maximal oxygen intake; uploads exercise data to your computer, allows five target heart rate zones, cleans your oven). Nike, Timex, Suunto, Reebok, Omron, Sigma, and Mio also make HRMs, and they all have their proponents. In my experience, Polar has the largest range of models and seems to dominate the triathlon groups I see. The supersimple models are a little too simplistic for any but the most beginning exerciser. The high-end models can be intimidating, but are incredibly useful if you want to train systematically. I go for the ones in the middle. Try getting a coded chest transmitter if you plan to work out in groups. The coded strap is linked to your wrist monitor and won't pick up interfering signals from other athletes.

The swankiest new HRM and general data toy I know of is the Garmin HRM and GPS (global positioning system). There's one for bikes and one for running. These bulky but cool devices give you all the heart rate and time functions of a regular HRM, plus they display your speed and the distance you've traveled using satellite data. Spendy, but so plush.

Sally says that the three biggest points of resistance to using an HRM are feeling uncomfortable with the chest strap, not knowing what the numbers mean, and just being unwilling to get the darn thing on and start the process. If you find yourself in any of these situations, there's help. Try different models of chest strap; try BodyGlide or Aquaphor to help the strap feel smoother on your skin; get help on the numbers from the good folks at the local store; and of course, just get out and do it.

SEPARATE MOVEMENT FROM WEIGHT LOSS

ANOTHER NUMBER THAT I urge you to pay less attention to is the one on the scale. If you take up physical activity with the primary aim of making that number shrink, I beg you to reconsider your priorities. It may happen, sure, but it won't necessarily happen just because you are exercising. Most people vastly underestimate the amount of exercise it takes to lose even a small amount of weight and vastly overestimate the calories they're "entitled to" after a workout.

The drive to reward oneself for effort expended with large amounts of succulent food is a powerful one (see Chapter 33). It probably even hearkens back to the primeval plains, where our ancestors chowed down on massive quantities of wildebeest after hours and hours of patiently jogging along after their prey. In our overfed society, with a dizzying variety of supersize meals awaiting us on every corner, it can be a challenge not to consume the caloric equivalent of a wildebeest after a relatively modest workout.

It's difficult to calibrate your food intake so that you fuel yourself adequately for your athletic endeavors but also get skinnier. For me, the only thing that's ever worked is following Weight Watchers diligently as I train. WW allows me to swap activity points for yummy foods and helps me keep track of energy in versus energy out. Otherwise I can train hard for a marathon or a half Ironman and gain weight while doing it. Not surprisingly, vigorous and sustained exercise makes me very hungry. Within thirty minutes to an hour after the workout, I'm ready to grab the squirming wildebeest and start eating it raw with a dash of sea salt and cracked pepper.

During the exercise session I have to consume calories so that I can keep going. For example, on a two-hour training run for a marathon, my HRM estimates that I burn about two thousand calories. But before starting I would gulp down about two hundred calories of a preexercise drink and then consume a hundred-calorie energy gel every thirty to forty-five minutes, adding up to as many as four hundred calories. Plus, I'd carry and consume another 150 calories' worth of sports drink. So when I look at my heart rate monitor and say to myself, "Whoa, dude, I've burned two thousand calories!" I have to remember that I've also taken in 750 calories already, approximately the equivalent of a Big Mac and a medium Coke. I also have to remember that the calorie burning part of the heart rate monitor is just an estimate.

Exercise does give you some leeway with dessert or French fries, but I don't think that should be the be-all and end-all of your motivation for doing it. I have talked to a lot of women who have taken up training for a big ol' endurance event and are upset with the fact that the pounds have not magically melted away. On the contrary, they are actually gaining weight. I'm like, "Well, do you feel stronger and more fit?" Yes, they do. "Do your clothes fit you better?" Yes, usually the clothes are getting looser. "Do you have more energy?" Yes. "Are you having fun?" Yes. "Then don't worry about the scale."

There are several factors at play in the phenomenon of weight gain through new habits of movement. One is the propensity to overfuel to compensate for the energy you're putting out. Most of us are not very good at hitting that balance. Another factor is that you may be building muscle and decreasing your percentage of body fat. Muscle is heavy stuff, compared to fat. A six-inch cube of lean muscle would be 22 percent heavier than a six-inch cube of fat. So your thighs could get skinnier but actually weigh more than they did before you took up your marathon training program, yoga, or dancing. Finally, as we discussed before, the equation of how many calories you actually burn per hour of activity changes as your body becomes more accustomed to the activity. In order to change the rate at which you burn calories, you have to vary your activities and keep your body from getting too comfortable.

Focusing on your weight as the desired outcome of your exercise limits you from appreciating all the other outcomes. You might sleep better, feel less tense, be nicer to your kids or coworkers, have better circulation, enjoy your food more, have more energy, feel better able to achieve your goals, and enjoy nature to a degree you'd never thought possible. Don't those outweigh (so to speak) the number on the scale? Uncouple your enjoyment of movement from your success at achieving the weight you think you should be at.

If you need to lose weight, and exercise is going to be a part of achieving that goal, that's great. Fine. Awesome, even. In fact, the National Weight Control Registry reports that most of the people who lose substantial amounts of weight (more than 30 pounds) and keep it off for five years or more (a tiny minority of people who try to lose weight) exercise vigorously for an average of an hour a day. Just remember two things: (1) exercise alone won't necessarily make you lose weight and (2) there are way more benefits to exercising than losing pounds.

Fitness and fun specialist Rocky Snyder says, "Most of my clients—probably 95 percent—come to me because they want to lose weight. But what happens instead is they get happy. They start moving and feeling stronger, then they start feeling better about themselves. Before long, they start seeing their bodies differently, with more pride, and they start eating differently. Some of my clients train with me for years and their basic body shapes haven't changed. But they do feel that they are in the best shape of their lives, and they're eating in a way that reflects the fact that each person is a miracle walking.

"I try to have people focus not so much on eating or not eating some particular food or food group, or even on having a specific eating plan, but on eating frequently, eating quality food, and on being conscious of what you eat. That is, paying attention to the fact that you are eating, what the food tastes and smells and looks like, where it comes from."

Rocky contends that regular movement, in a variety of arenas that you find fun, can make you happy. And not just in a superficial way, but seeing the spark of the divine in yourself and the world all around you. Beats the heck out of cabbage soup.

SEE MOVEMENT
AS A PRIVILEGE

SIMPLY **BEING ABLE** to move your body around is something that should make you feel awed and grateful every day. And not in a nagging type of way: "Oh, you should be grateful for those canned green beans; think of all the starving children in Africa who don't have anything to eat." More on a larger scale: "You should be grateful for air, and water and trees and chocolate." Just as Rocky said in the last chapter, you are a miracle walking.

Go to any large gym or health club, and look at the rows and rows of sweating automatons on the Stairmasters, treadmills, ellipticals, and stationary bikes. You'll see lots of iPods, magazines, and books. Lots of grim concentration. It's not just an indoor phenomenon, though. I see plenty of runners out there who look like they're enduring the most inventive tortures of the Spanish Inquisition or, worse, a three-hour meeting complete with a dull PowerPoint that you can't read because the stupid font is too small. Cyclists too. And hikers, aerobicizers, even rollerbladers! I mean, how can you turn roller skating into drudgery? That ain't right.

There are going to be days when you don't look forward to exercise, but you have to remember that it's just great to be able to move at all. Try and remember how bad you felt, how stiff and tired and sluggish you felt before you started moving on a regular basis.

Kyle is a wonderful man who belongs to my triathlon club. He's one of the best triathletes in the country in his mid-forties age-group, so he's been doing it for a while. He's really, really good at his sports, and if you saw him zipping by you on the track you might think, "Oh, that guy's really fast and talented; he must look down on my slow fat self and think mean thoughts." But you would be totally wrong. Kyle almost always wins his age-group in our local races or comes in second, so I've cheered him on many a podium. Usually you have to wait around a long time to get your award, so once I said to him in jest, "Hey, Kyle, doesn't it get old getting up on that podium all the time and getting your picture taken?" He looked at me intently and said, "No, never. It's a privilege and an honor to be able to train and race." And I immediately realized that he was absolutely right. When our bodies are healthy and able to move, it's a gift.

Think of someone you know, maybe someone in your family, a friend, a coworker, who's been through a debilitating injury or illness. Or maybe you've been there. Heart surgery, car crash, broken leg, cancer, Lyme disease, stroke. If you've been through that, think back on how much you would have given to be able to go for a run or a bike ride, even if it was hard and made you sweat and pant. If it was someone you knew, you might have suffered just watching him or her in pain, bored, stiff, wishing that person you cared about could move around, just get up and go walk around the block. Not being able to move? Now that's drudgery.

TRAIN YOUR BRAIN TO BE A POSITIVE ENERGY GENERATOR

THIS MAY SOUND as corny as those motivational posters on office walls. I used to be skeptical of "the power of positive thinking" and repeating affirmations and stuff like that. I just kept thinking of Stuart Smalley and "I'm good enough, I'm smart enough, and doggone it, people like me!"

In my second season as a triathlete, however, my attitude about positive thinking shifted somewhat. I signed up for private coaching with Lisa Engles because I had registered for a half Ironman and I was scared witless. Lisa generated weekly training plans, we talked on the phone, and all her charges gathered once a week for small group workouts—track intervals or transition drills on how to take off a wetsuit as quickly as possible, that sort of thing.

I had been making great progress. I had dropped weight over the preceding year, and I had followed Lisa's training plans closely. I was getting faster and faster, and was getting solidly into the middle of the pack, which was a real achievement considering where I had started. But I had never broken the ten-minute mile running pace, and it seemed as huge a barrier to me as the four-minute mile had to runners before Roger Bannister ran it in 3:59.4 in 1954.

As we headed into race season, Lisa started emphasizing the "mental training" aspect of triathlon. I rolled my eyes. We were supposed to come up with personal affirmations that started with "I," like "I slice through the water like a knife" or "I am powerful on hills." Being the smartass that I am, I started popping out with "I float in the water like a dead whale" and "I am faster than a stalled car." Finally Lisa got me to buy into the program by telling me that the affirmations would work whether my conscious mind believed in them or not. I thought, okay, what the heck. What harm's it going to do? Lisa's coaching had been working in other areas, so I decided to give this a shot too.

I came up with some affirmations that I could say to myself (though I could never bring myself to look in the mirror and say them out loud), and I practiced thinking them. "I have trained for a personal best," and "I am a strong runner. I get stronger as the race goes on." I even came up with the catchy, "I am fast; I have fun, as I float along the run." On the way to my second race of the year, I actually got pretty pumped up. I chanted my affirmations out loud, pounding out a rhythm on the steering wheel as I let loose. This is why I do not generally car-pool to races.

I had a good swim and a solid bike ride. The last couple of miles on the bike are mostly uphill, so my legs were a little tired as I headed out onto Uvas Road for the run. But I focused on my run cadence, on relaxing my shoulders, and on breathing deeply and evenly, and soon that wobbly feeling went away. I hit the mile 1 marker in just around ten minutes and felt pleased, since the first mile is the hardest in any tri. Mile 2 was similar, but at mile 3 my split time was 9:51. With two miles to go, I had a chance to average under–ten minute miles. "I am fast; I have fun, as I float along the run," I thought. "I have trained for a personal best. I am ready." I pushed myself to pick up the pace, while keeping my shoulders relaxed, my feet moving at 170 steps per minute, and the breathing coordinated with the steps. At mile 4 I was still under pace, with one mile to go. Lisa found me at about the half-mile mark and yelled encouragement. I cruised up the last little rise and around the corner feeling like a real runner. I finished the five miles in forty-eight minutes and change, by far my fastest run ever.

At my next race, which was longer and harder, I lowered my average run time to 9:17 per mile. And it didn't even hurt. I had worked my affirmations extremely hard before and during the race, but I had also trained diligently and consistently.

The mental training works great to aid your performance, but only if you also do the physical preparation. And you have to keep your affirmations realistic. If your fastest time ever is an eight-minute mile, you can't repeat, "I'm going to average five-minute miles" ten thousand times and expect it to happen. In fact, stay away from specific numbers altogether. Be more general: "I am strong," or "I have fun with every mile I run." If you are coming up to an event where you really want to peak and you've done the homework physically, I think it's okay to affirm to yourself, "I am ready to have a breakthrough performance."

It's okay to do frivolous affirmations, as long as they have a serious core. During my marathon training, I was in a phase where I listened to the happy (and poignant) island tunes of

Israel Kamakawiwo'ole, or Brudda Iz, a master of modern and traditional Hawaiian music. So while I jogged along on my multihour training runs, I'd make up lyrics of my own to one of my favorite Iz songs. Like this:

> *Ha'ina mai kapuana [Let everybody hear my story]*
> *I'm a marathon runner*
> *I'm having fun in the sun*
> *I kick okole [butt] when I run*

It probably sounds more poetic in Hawaiian. Anyway, the point is that my lyrics were silly and serious too. I was utterly serious about finishing that marathon, and about having fun while I did both the training and the race. And I did.

And you can too.

ADVANCED BRAIN TRAINING
WITH GUEST STAR LISA ENGLES

Lisa says:

"Ask yourself powerful questions. Ask yourself what your fears are: there are several that are common to everybody like 'I don't deserve to succeed'; or 'I'm just not good at this.' Then identify the secondary benefits for holding on to your limiting beliefs. Does believing this make you right and others wrong? Is it an ego thing? Is it a way to get out of responsibility? Does it make you feel safe? It can be scary to change. Not one person in this world doesn't have limiting belief. And everyone holds onto them with the illusion that the belief is benefiting them.

"Ask, What if? What if I could have fun doing this? What would that be like? Or what if I were really good at sports? What would my training be like?

"As an example, I was working with athlete who said, 'I want to run a 10k in forty minutes.' By all his benchmark tests it was obvious that he should be able to do this. His limiting belief was that he was genetically incapable of being as fast as other people. Then he rationalized his slower times in races by saying, 'I'm just doing this for fun.' But that was hiding a fear of failing at something he really wanted to do. Then if he failed at it, it didn't matter. What was the benefit to him of holding onto the belief, 'I'm not capable'? He could keep believing, 'I don't have to try as hard. I don't have to do the track workout; I don't have to do all the training.'"

So ask yourself, What if I were capable of running a marathon? What would I do? How would I carry myself? What else would I believe?

What if?

BE YOUR OWN SUPERHERO

WHEN I WAS a kid, back when woolly mammoths roamed the glacial plains, people didn't wear shiny tights and form-fitting unitards. There was no Lycra, no spandex, no neoprene. Only superheroes wore that kind of stuff on TV or in the movies and in comic books. Their outfits hugged their bodies in a fantastic way. The fabrics were sleek and glossy, part and parcel of the superheroes' powers.

The only real people who looked like superheroes to me were the intrepid explorers of Jacques Cousteau's underwater team. In their chic little black wetsuits and mysterious scuba tanks, they clearly had powers that mere mortals did not. I envied them. Later on, in the 1980s, elite athletes started to appear in their exotic technical fabrics. I remember some downhill skiers wearing neon-trimmed suits at Sarajevo, and then in 1988, Alberto Tomba, "La Bomba," went super form fitting. Then swimmers started wearing the full bodysuits made out of "FastSkin," a superstretchy fabric with little ridges that imitate the texture of shark skin, and other space-age duds.

Also in the 1980s, stretchy bike shorts and leggings first became available in mass-market retail outlets, giving normal folks an opportunity to dress like superheroes. I remember my first pair of shiny running tights, slinky, black, and adhering to my legs like a coat of paint. I felt faster, as if I were passing through the air unnoticed by the forces of friction. When I got my first wetsuit years later, that feeling of magically enhanced ability returned.

Feeling like a superhero, though, is about more than form-fitting fabrics and the courage to wear them. It's also about recognizing that your ordinary powers are actually as cool as superpowers, if you just develop them. Batman wasn't even a superhero, technically speaking. He had no superpowers. He just had an unstoppable commitment to justice and crime fighting.

When you tap into your own unstoppable commitment to do everything within your power to follow your dreams, that makes you a superhero too. When you're committed, you are unstoppable. You can conquer the world. They can line up the Joker, the Penguin, Lex Luthor, the Green Goblin, and the Mirror Master against you, and you can pile-drive them over, one by one or all at the same time. I'm not kidding about this. No one can stop you from achieving your dreams, athletic or otherwise, if you make a flat-out, full-on commitment to them.

The problem is that most of the time most of us aren't willing to do the things that full commitment would demand. We're not willing to take a three-month unpaid leave from our jobs and put our bikes on the road in Anacortes, armed only with cycling route maps, two panniers full of gear, and an aim to take that bike all the way to Connecticut. We're not willing to keep watching our food intake and training consistently, even on business trips, until we've lost 163 pounds and are preparing for our first Ironman. But some people are, and I've watched them follow their will and their commitment to incredible places.

My own commitment to my dreams has wavered and flickered; I've ceased to control my eating, I've eased off my training, and I've put other things ahead of triathlon. That doesn't make me a bad person, it just means that I've been trying to balance various priorities in my life, and athletics haven't always been number one. But I know, from watching my friends, that if I ever really emulate them and give my all to my dream, no matter what it takes, I can achieve it, and so can you. And isn't that just a little super?

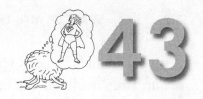

GET HELP WHEN
YOU NEED IT

THE ROAD TO athletehood is not an easy one. Sometimes you need a doctor. Or a coach. Or a chiropractor. Or just a helping hand with all your stuff.

You don't have to become an athlete all on your own. You can (see Chapter 30), but you don't have to. There's a lot of help out there, and I encourage you to take advantage of it. Getting help doesn't make you weaker, it makes you stronger. What kind of help, you ask?

Sport-Specific Help. This can come in a variety of forms, from an informative and detailed book to a club of like-minded individuals to a coach who can devise a whole training program for you. Some sports require a whole community to figure out. It's really hard to do volleyball on your own, for example, while distance running is something you can tackle as an individual. But even for loner sports that don't involve a lot of obvious technique or expensive facilities, there are some advantages to getting information. Even with running, you can learn how to set up your workouts for maximum progress and minimum trauma; how to pace yourself, how to breathe (seriously!), what your heart rate means, and all kinds of technical goodies.

Social Help.   Not so much help, but maybe support. Tips and tricks from a pack of folks who've latched on to the same sport you have. You can find your sports soul mates online or in person, or both. I'm very partial to a group of Weight Watchers members, both actively losing and maintaining their weight loss (for years, dammit! How do they do it?), who do triathlons and post daily on the Weight Watchers bulletin boards. I'm also very fond of my local Silicon Valley Triathlon Club. I've learned all kinds of things from SVTC, from how to change a tire to blister-avoidance techniques. If I want folks to work out with, I can almost always find them, and it's great to see my buds at races and feel like part of the crew. Social pressures can help you stay on track with your workout regiment. It's a lot easier to blow off that early morning workout if it's just you, but if your friends are out at the bike shop parking lot waiting for you, you'll think hard before you hit that snooze button for the eighth time.

Inspirational Help.   Mostly what I learn from my club and my Weight Watchers buddies, though, is inspiration. I see people who have jobs twice as hard as mine, who have kids, who have medical issues, who have every obstacle you can imagine—and yet they are out there training, racing, having a great time, enjoying each other's company, and enjoying the week-in, week-out process of perfecting their imperfectly athletic selves. Some of my fellow SVTC-ers are way more perfectly athletic than others. They qualify for national and world championships at various distances in various age-groups, and they go out and ac-quit themselves pretty darn well. But they always have a friendly greeting for a slug like me. That in itself is pretty inspirational.

Musculo-Skeletal Help. If you're prone to nagging injuries or you just got your first one, it's good to have someone handy to help get you back on your feet again. These angels with special tables come in many guises: massage therapist, chiropractor, or physical therapist. Find one who is willing to learn your body and how it works: that nagging pain in the sacro-iliac joint on the right side; the way the muscle at the top of your leg seems to twist itself forward and around; the shoulder that always hurts after a long swim workout. You may need occasional doses of ultrasound or electro-stim. A good musculo-skeletal health pro will give you exercises and stretches to do to keep you from reinjuring yourself. Do the exercises. And when the injury quits hurting, keep doing the exercises.

Mechanical Help. Depending on your sport, you may or may not have equipment that needs tweaking. If you have anything with moving parts, though, it's good to have the pros check the gear out. Get your bike tuned up and checked, for example. Or your skis, or your tennis racket. If you're returning to your youth as a power-hitting softball player, hang with the folks at the store that specializes in bats, gloves, spikes, and batting hel-mets. Maybe you're swinging the wrong length bat or the wrong weight. Maybe you'd be better off with different shoes. Get to know the experts and learn as much as you can about the equipment you depend on. On a bike, a misadjustment of just a quarter inch in the handlebars or saddle position can cause mysterious and debilitating pain. You might need help to spot that.

Logistical Help.   Sometimes you may need support when it comes to just getting everything done. Can you delegate household chores or errands to family members? Can you delegate cooking to the supermarket rotisserie chicken people once a week? Can you do a "freezer filling" party with two or three other busy athletes—cook a huge mess of some tasty, reasonably healthy dinner, split it into freezable portions, and share it with your cooking partners? Can you get someone in to clean the house once a month?

You may also want logistical help for a big event. Marathoner Russ and his wife Michelle have a good system going when he runs marathons. He designates intersections for her to wait at with supplies of energy gels, drinks, even fresh socks. Michelle follows the map, finds her spot around the estimated time of arrival, and makes the handoff, along with a loving smooch. The smooch helps a lot.

Moral Support Help.   Even if your nearest and dearest don't need to hand you a fresh water bottle or retape your ankles between fights, you still need them to love you for what you're doing in your sport. You are an athlete! You are a superhero! You rock! And whatever it is you're doing, it's pretty amazing. Moral support comes in all different guises. My husband rarely wants to get up early and watch me race, and that's cool. But he shows up for the big ones, even though standing up for a long time makes his back hurt. And after my little local races, he comes out as soon as he hears my car pull in, to help me unload my bike and my piles of sweaty, salty stuff. And he never complains when those piles of sweaty race gear are still lying out on the patio on Wednesday because I haven't had the energy or time to stick them in the wash. Now that's moral support.

SECTION VI

SEVEN PRACTICES TO INSPIRE YOUR SPIRIT

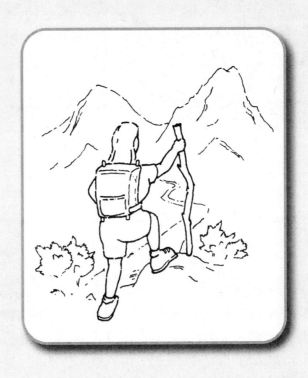

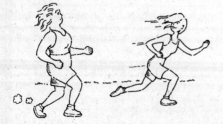

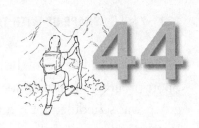

BE A PIT BULL

PIT BULLS HAVE had a lot of bad press. Lots of cities want to outlaw them; unscrupulous characters breed pit bulls and pit bull crosses under cruel conditions and treat the dogs badly, and sometimes one of those dogs goes nuts and mauls someone.

I'm not saying that you should go nuts and maul someone. The pit bull was bred for absolute, never-surrender tenacity in the service of bullbaiting, a sport that was later outlawed, but the tenacity remains. And that tenacity is what I want you to find in yourself. Chapter 42 talked about the power of commitment. This is more about hanging on to that commitment when circumstances test it. You've got your jaws clamped on to the pants leg of your dreams, but you get shaken around, tossed and buffeted by life. You have setbacks, you have bad weather, you have injuries. You want to quit. You want to lie on the couch. You want to let go. But as a pit bull, you don't let go. Ever.

If you don't like the image of yourself as a pit bull on the pants leg of your dreams, pick another dog.

Dan Sauers has been the coach of my tri club's New to the Sport program on and off for years. One weekend in March, our group was scheduled for a run, and the forecast was for temperatures in the forties, high winds, and rain squalls. Dan wrote the group this e-mail the day before:

Be prepared for blustery, cool conditions. But don't be deterred! This is a great opportunity to not only get in a good physical workout but to score BIG mental bonus points!! After you've done all the physical preparation, it really comes down to how tough your head is! Doing your planned workouts regardless of what Mother Nature throws at you is one place you get tough. So, if the weather is cold, windy, wet or all three—no negative thoughts, use the challenge to your advantage.

I am picturing a park replete with acres of grassy hillocks. A creek-fed pond with ducks and geese, and a loon. Majestic conifers and robust broadleaf trees, squirrels and jays. A light breeze swirls leaves beneath outstretched boughs. A young girl, a boy, a little white and rust-brown terrier and a sock with one end tied in a knot. What a game of tug-of-war they're having! Grrrrr rrR. That little terrier has locked onto that sock and claimed it for his own. Grrr rrrr. So much so, that when the boy lifts the sock high, that feisty little dog stays right with it, clear off the ground. GrrRR rrrr not a thought of letting go . . . ggrrr RR rrr. Be that little dog.

I love this little motivational vignette. Dan guides us through the imagery of cold, blustery weather attacking unwary runners and then he takes us beyond, into the pastoral park with the kids and the little brown-and-white terrier. It turns from work and the need to gain mental toughness into a game, kids playing with a dog. Dan transforms the image of never-give-up tenacity from something grim to something playful. The dog is not holding on because he has to; he wants to. He's smaller than the sock wielder, but he's not daunted.

If you look at a rough spot in your training schedule as a game of tug-of-war in the park, it suddenly seems a lot less threatening. Your rough spot might be small—a storm forecast for the day of your long run—or it might be a knee operation, a change in your work schedule, a family member who needs care. You need to lock onto the sock. Even if your feet get lifted off the ground, your focus has to be the sock, whether it is your marathon, your triathlon, or a trek in Nepal. You can make it happen one day. Maybe not today or next week, but someday, as long as you don't let go of the sock.

More perspective from the indomitable Rebecca, triathlete, volleyball player, and activewear activist from Chapter 2 on never, ever letting go:

> My right shoulder has hurt for seventeen or eighteen years, and two years ago, I tweaked my left shoulder during a tough volley-ball game, so now that shoulder hurts too whenever I play. All this and I have played volleyball for thirty-six years. I can give in to my stiffness and pain, or I can take my ibuprofen and go out and play. It's an addiction; the game just gets in your blood and stays there. It's important to find something active in life you enjoy, whether you're good at it, or it is just good with you. Volleyball is therapy; being active is therapy. Winning the match doesn't really matter. Playing well, being active, and having a good time does. There's just nothing like being able to

stuff block a player half your age. And there's nothing like being almost forty-six years old, and being able to jump nineteen inches off the floor, reach high, and kill the spike, slamming the ball into a big empty space on the court. And to know, even though I can't move well in the back court anymore, that I'm inspiring younger women, that's magic.

Be that little dog.

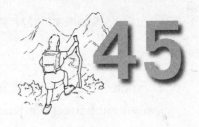

GET HIGH
(INTO THE MOUNTAINS)

OR GO TO the desert, the Florida Everglades, the Boundary Waters of northern Minnesota, even Alaska. Why? Because going outside is good, and going way outside, into some extreme environment, is even better. I believe strongly that the lessons learned out in the wilderness are life changing for anyone, and fundamentally important for people who want to emerge from the habits of couch potato sloth and into the Way of Shameless Fitness.

If you are ready to walk the way with me, then assume the lotus position and listen carefully, diverting your mind from the pain in your knees. As I have been saying in various ways, becoming an athlete involves developing your physical strength, flexibility, endurance, and sport-specific skills. It also involves developing yourself mentally: your focus, your ability to interpret your body's effort, your resiliency, your self-confidence, your planning skills, and your determination. So why wouldn't a six- or seven-day excursion into an environment that's physically and mentally challenging be a perfect way to develop your Way of Shameless Fitness? Well, it would. Duh.

I was an imperfect outdoorswoman before I became an imperfect endurance athlete. When I fled graduate school in search of a life of more adventure, I fell into a job with a fledgling nonprofit called Project RAFT (Russians and Americans for Teamwork). The idea was that getting Russians (Soviets, at that time) into rafts with Americans and sending them together down a whitewater river in the wilderness would teach them the necessity of teamwork for a common goal, leaving them more interested in peace and less in mutual nuclear annihilation. The founders of Project RAFT were world-class raft guides who spoke no Russian. I spoke Russian rather well for an American but had no rafting experience.

Over the course of the next five years, I spent weeks at a time living in tents, getting soaking wet, hauling heavy bags and packs, cooking over open fires and propane, fixing rafts as darkness fell, and dealing with mosquitoes the size of Siberian eagles. I used Russian bug repellent so harsh it stripped the varnish off a guitar, and I am here to tell the tale.

In isolated incidents, I ate raw reindeer brains in northern Siberia; sprained my ankle and got the river crud on a single day in Zambia; sank up to my hips in swamp mud; busted a handmade reindeer-drawn sled by running it into a tree; and got bitten on the coochie by a giant horsefly while playing the role of the Statue of Liberty in a wilderness Fourth of July pageant. While I never achieved the level of outdoor skill of my compadres who spent their formative years climbing, kayaking, trekking, and cross-country skiing, I became pretty much at ease in a lot of different environments. I also learned to drink vodka in quantities I no longer consider prudent.

Besides that lesson, though, I learned a lot of other things that later stood me in good stead as an imperfect but usually good-humored athlete:

It's Not About the Gear.   This one I learned from the Russians. We Americans came cruising into the Altai Mountains of Siberia with our high-tech self-bailing rafts, lightweight plastic paddles, drysuits, helmets, and dry boxes, planning to show the Russians how to raft. As it happened the Russians had designed hand-built catamaran rafts that were lighter, more collapsible, and way more maneuverable than our big old beasts. They were harder to rig and maintain, but they worked amazingly well in gnarly whitewater, and our new Siberian friends had built them in their apartments out of old truck inner tubes and lengths of nylon. The Russians made homemade drysuits out of rubber and used stolen Aeroflot life jackets and scavenged hockey helmets. Their paddles were often aluminum blades with a birch sapling stripped and shoved into a lugged handle. And these guys had at least as much fun as we did.

Laughing Is Better Than Whining.   Once I was part of an international teambuilding exercise in the Sierras in winter. We had a cozy lodge, but we spent all day out on cross-country skis, trying to follow complicated topographic maps and hit a bunch of checkpoints. I was the second least experienced cross-country skier in the group, and my Russian friend Sergei accurately but tactlessly likened my technique to a cow on ice. I fell over a lot. The least experienced skier was a young outdoorsman from Japan. He fell over constantly, like every fifty feet. But he bounced back up and laughed like crazy, shaking snow out of his hair. When I fell down, I would struggle to my feet, swearing and grunting, and say something like, "Who the hell had this stupid idea?" Needless to say, Aida-san was a lot more popular than me by the end of the day.

Sometimes Whining Is Okay Too.   If the only way you're going to get through the freezing cold day in the boat, the endless uphill over a steep pass, the long slog down a trail overgrown with jumping cholla cactus is to whine, then go ahead. Hopefully you'll be with friends who understand you and know that you're just blowing off steam. Otherwise, explain up front that you just need to whine a little to blow off steam, and you'll be better soon. Even if you don't think you will.

Suffering Ends.   I have been uncomfortable, in distress, and even in pain on outdoor expeditions all over the world. I've had blisters the size of tangerines, sprained ankles, battered feet, sunburns, stomach upsets, and bronchitis. I've been way too hot, way too cold, way too hungry, and way too chafed. I've lost multiple toenails as a result of backpacking. I've had neck spasms in a Siberian reindeer herders' camp. I've had a sprained ankle and simultaneous vomiting and diarrhea on a Zambian riverbank. But none of it had permanent consequences. My second toenails don't look quite as nice as they used to but it's nothing a pedicure won't disguise. Suffering ends eventually, and when it does you have a heck of a story to tell.

It's All About the Feet.   Last summer, I went backpacking in Sequoia National Park with my old friend Anne. Unfortunately, I hadn't been on a recent hike with my backpacking boots before we hit the trail. I was only into the second day on an easy trail when I realized the boots had passed their prime.

The midsoles had completely lost their ability to support and to absorb shock. It took me a while to realize why my feet hurt so much, my knees ached, my back was stiff, and my hips were complaining bitterly: my boots were old. When you weigh a lot and then carry a forty-pound pack, you better have boots that work. Even if your weight is normal, you still need boots that are designed to support and cushion your feet against the extra load and the rocks, roots, and downhills of the trail. Even if you're not carrying a heavy pack, remember that without happy feet, you can't have a happy hike. Anne informs me that every time we came to a break, whether our lunchtime stop or our break for camp, I hurled my pack down and let loose a resounding F-bomb. At night I would get cramps in my legs, back, and even my stomach muscles. So make sure you have your feet taken care of. It was one of the most beautiful hikes ever, but physically it was the most miserable. All because I didn't take an hour for a test hike. In the immortal words of Homer, "Doh!"

You Can Face Down Your Fears. Anne is a professor of (mostly) obscure film, a mother of three girls, a novelist, an accomplished violinist, a songwriter, and a poet. It's no easy thing for her to get away from her obligations for a week and head into the mountains. But she does, and here's one of the reasons why:

> We were slogging our way into the Sierras from the eastern side, walking up along a reservoir, our poor lowlander lungs gasping for air. On the other side of the water was an intensely steep hillside of scree, about one degree shy of an outright cliff, all pebbles and rocks and scary stuff—and across that cliff-like frozen landslide of a slope ran the thinnest of lines. "Hey," said

Jayne, "That's the trail we come out on at the end of our trip." And my heart just about stopped.

I love mountains more than anything, and backpacking's my very most favorite activity in the world, but I have deep unwillingness to risk falling down cliffs to my death. I'm afraid of heights. I hate having to traverse steep patches of snow, and scree is even worse. (Think of all the bruises you'd get as you fell to your death!) I looked at that line across the cliff and thought, no way. I spent the next five days thinking no way, no way, no way! My secret conviction was that when we got to that awful place on the last day, I was going to end up shaking so hard I'd have to turn around and go back the lo-o-ong way. And here's the thing: when seen up close, the trail was not just a line across a cliff. It was an actual trail, a kind of solid, comforting trail with ample space even for my large feet. And instead of trembling and turning around, I found myself walking along (eyes forward!) almost like a normal person, and inside my heart was laughing. The joke was on me, and I was glad of it!

Take a couple of weeks off and go somewhere extreme. Do something that requires you to travel at least partially under your own power for days at a time, out where you can't run to the store for a pint of Ben & Jerry's when you feel down. It doesn't have to be the Iditarod, but it should be something that makes you a little nervous, and hopefully in a place you find attractive and/or interesting. When you get back, you'll find that your hour-long workout is a lot easier than it used to be.

THE LOWDOWN: MAKING THE WORDS REAL

Are you one of those people who don't camp? Well, then, don't camp, if you're truly committed to the non-outdoorsy life. But if the idea intrigues you at all, here are some things to think about.

Backpacking or car camping?   Car camping is great: you have a huge cooler full of food, lots of chairs, a roomy tent, a campfire ring, marshmallows, the works. There are often flush toilets, sometimes even showers. Parks and preserves can be crowded and noisy, but they can be a great way to get your feet wet in the forest, desert, pine barrens, or hills. You can make some great day hikes from a base camp with your car too. Backpacking requires a lot more organization and should be undertaken initially with an experienced companion. If you don't have an experienced companion, there are outdoors clubs and classes that will help you get outfitted and take you on overnight outings for a modest fee. Backpacking gets you into the part of the outdoors that really makes you think, "Gee, I'm a puny little human in the middle of all this." And that can be very rewarding. Think about your tolerance for getting dirty before you make your decision.

Or some other kind of adventure?   Multiday expeditions on boats can get you into places that you can't get to any other way, which is pretty amazing. Again, you can pay people to guide you places on boats, and unless you have some pretty hard-core boating friends, I recommend you do so. There are also mountain bike tours that can get you pretty far outdoors. You can pack into a remote place on a mule and save your hiking energies for exploring around the remote place.

Gear.   If, unlike me, you do not like buying lots of sports equipment, you are not excluded from the outdoors. Rentals are

continues

The Lowdown: Making the Words Real *continued*

usually available from local outfitters, along with a guided tour and general advice. For example, if you're going on a canoe tour, don't use a down sleeping bag. Down clumps when it gets wet, and you get cold. Synthetic fibers work better for water-borne adventure.

Planning your trip. How much time do you have to spend out in the wild? How long do you think you can last? Will you be able to buy more food at your campground or nearby town, or do you need to haul it in with you? Do you have good maps of the area? What are the weather conditions likely to be? What are the potential hazards—heat, cold, poison oak/ivy, mosquitoes?

Boots. Have I said enough about boots? They don't need to cost an arm and a leg, but they need to fit, be comfortable, and support your feet. I recommend you not buy hiking boots for $29.99 at your local Shoe Blowout Warehouse.

46

CARE PASSIONATELY ABOUT YOUR ABSURD ENDEAVORS

HEY, **WHO ARE** you calling absurd? Well, you, to start off with. But also me, and all of us who are striving and straining and putting huge amounts of time and energy into achieving very middling results, as measured by "objective" standards like "winning" and "losing" and "finishing in the top 90 percent of all racers." I mean, this is silly stuff we're doing here. And I invite you to embrace that silliness wholeheartedly. Embracing silliness, though, does not mean downplaying the importance of your efforts. Your work and play in becoming an athlete is a journey that affects your life, and quite possibly the lives of many other people. I have met and corresponded with all kinds of people whose pursuit of a sport has inspired them to change jobs, write books, raise huge amounts of funds for charity, coach others, and become community leaders advocating for health and fitness.

But please don't lose your sense of humor over this stuff. Remember, ain't nobody paying us to do this. Sometimes I see this T-shirt at endurance events: "Pain Is Weakness Leaving the Body." Well, maybe. But geez, do ya have to be so Navy SEALS-ish about it? Let's not be focusing on pain and weakness and strength and domination. I prefer the T-shirt that reads "Will Run for Food." Even though it contradicts my advice to stop rewarding yourself for exercise with food, I still like it. It's funny.

A wise Hungarian psychologist named Mihalyi Csikszentmihalyi once wrote, "Buddhists advise us to 'act always as if the future of the universe depended on what you did, while laughing at yourself for thinking that whatever you do makes any difference.' This serious playfulness makes it possible to be both engaged and carefree at the same time."

Dude. That is like, so totally true. What has worked best for me in my athletic career and my life (and if you haven't figured out by now that the two are inextricably linked, go back and read the book again from the beginning) has been a passionate dedication to my goals with a parallel determination to laugh at myself every step of the way.

If you're not fully engaged, then you're not going to get the maximum satisfaction out of your sport. Being engaged, being committed, means that you pay attention to what you're doing. You're consistent, except for those times when your close attention tells you that you need to mix things up and be inconsistent for a while. You challenge yourself at the level where you can experience progress rather than frustration. You care about what you're doing, whether it's climbing Charles Mound or Mount Whitney, wheeling and jabbing in cardio kickboxing class, sailing to Hawaii, swimming from Alcatraz to San Francisco, or digging a volleyball. Because if you don't care, why bother?

So care passionately about getting the most out of your sport. But don't get so caught up in the numbers, your goals, the people around you, or your own idea of what you should be doing and how you should be doing it, that you forget to laugh.

What you are doing in your sport has no importance in the grand scheme of things. A hundred years from now, your greatest athletic achievement will rest in oblivion, along with other people's achievements. Although that may sound depressing to some, I find it liberating. It frees me up to make mistakes, go out on a limb, cheer and shout and make an idiot of myself as I stand on a chilly beach at dawn, waiting to charge into the waves with a hundred neoprene-clad strangers. It frees me to enjoy the sights and sounds and smells of my sport because I know I'm doing this for the experience of the present moment as well as for my dreams and goals.

I know a guy in Fairbanks, Alaska, who goes by the name of Bad Bob. He's a very amiable person, not particularly bad in any sense of the word, except perhaps that he is an absolute badass at cross-country skiing. He competes at an international level in the "masters" age-group, and he and a buddy hold the record for skiing the renowned Iditarod trail. That's about 1,100 miles from Anchorage to Nome, with subzero temperatures, howling winds, unpredictable snow conditions, and stretches of absolute desolation that can strike fear into your heart just watching them on TV. But that's not what Bob talked about as he sat with Tim and me over plates of ribs and coleslaw. For Bad Bob, spending three weeks out in the freezing cold with a heavy backpack on skis was just plain fun. And in his soft-spoken, understated way, he conveyed both that he was intensely proud of the accomplishment and that he found the whole endeavor to be pretty funny.

So if Bad Bob takes his accomplishments lightly, I think it would be fitting for all of us to see the absurd side of our efforts while acknowledging how much they mean to us.

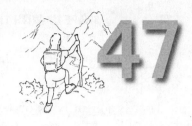

FIND THE FLOW

WHAT IS FLOW, and why do you want to find it? It has nothing to do with your bodily fluids, so you can relax on that score. Flow, as applied to athletic endeavors, is that almost mystical state where time and effort seem to disappear. Your body is moving easily, almost of its own volition. You're aware of your arms and legs and core muscles in motion, but you don't have a sense of working hard to make them move. Your mind is clear and light, focused on the matter at hand but free of anxiety and tension. All the work, all the hours of practice and training, mental preparation, affirmations, and figuring out logistics are part of your being. You are in the zone, and you are having a peak performance.

Sounds pretty good, huh? Damn straight it is. And it is pretty much the definition of fun. There's nowhere else you'd rather be, and there's nothing else you'd rather be doing than what you're doing right now. The trick is finding that flow. If it were easier to find, the roads would be clogged with bicycles, and the trails gridlocked with runners and hikers. You wouldn't be able to keep people from exercising; the flow feels so awesome when it happens.

There's a great book on flow that I recommend to all imperfect athletes. Unfortunately, the author's name is almost guaranteed to make you choke and stammer, which is not a good start for finding flow. He is psychology professor Mihaly Csikszentmihaly. My best shot at pronouncing it is "Mee-HAI CHIK-shent-mee-HAI," but all you Hungarians out there, please feel free to correct me. The book is called *Flow: The Psychology of Optimal Experience*, and it offers a lot of good and very readable information about what flow is and how to tap into it, not just in athletics but in your everyday life.

Until you can get down to your local bookstore and grab a copy of *Flow*, I've got a few of Csikszentmihalyi's key points here, along with some observations of my own. But do check out the Csik-man; he rocks.

Flow Means Active Happiness.   "It is the full involvement of flow, rather than happiness, that makes for excellence in life. We can be happy experiencing the passive pleasure of a rested body, warm sunshine, or the contentment of a serene relationship, but this kind of happiness is dependent on favorable external circumstances. The happiness that follows flow is of our own making, and it leads to increasing complexity and growth in consciousness." What I like about this is that happiness is defined as something that you create out of your own intense involvement in an activity.

It's Not So Important What the Activity Is.   "Flow generally occurs when a person is doing his or her favorite activity—

gardening, listening to music, bowling, cooking a good meal. It also occurs when driving, talking to friends, and surprisingly often at work." I myself have often found flow—losing track of time, becoming so absorbed in my activity that I was unaware of hunger or thirst (which is unusual for me, trust me)—in the process of creating multiyear budgets for state or federal grant applications. This is not something I choose to do in my leisure time, but as my work life has progressed, I have become increasingly aware that I actually kind of dig doing budgets. I also find flow riding my bike, swimming laps, kicking a foot bag, and, more rarely, running. Not surprisingly, people report that sports is one of the best ways to get into a flow state. Other situations with well-determined goals and set techniques like crafts, music, and games work too. MC says, "Flow tends to occur when a person faces a clear set of goals that require appropriate responses." So if your goal is to ride your bike fifty miles, that's clear. And the appropriate response is also clear. Figure out a route, get on your bike, set your bike computer, and start pedaling.

Flow Is About Learning and Mastering Skills.   MC also says that "flow also happens when a person's skills are fully involved in overcoming a challenge that is just about manageable, so it acts as a magnet for learning new skills and increasing challenges. If challenges are too low, one gets back to flow by increasing them. If challenges are too great, one can return to the flow state by learning new skills." This is a perfect description for the process of becoming proficient in a sport, whether it's squash or running or street luge. You're always in a cycle of testing your skills, pushing yourself, easing off and consolidating your gains, then looking at new challenges.

Watching TV Is Not Conducive to Finding Flow.　It ranks lowest on the list of leisure activities that induce flow. Work, no matter how you claim to hate it, is much more likely to get you into a flow state than TV is. Not that we don't all need a little down time with our favorite shows, but it's a low-investment, low-return leisure strategy. Getting into flow requires investment of attention and energy, but it returns your investment many times over. In fact, people who frequently read books report getting into a flow state more often than people who don't—not just during reading but during other activities too.

"To learn to control attention, any skill or discipline one can master on one's own will serve: meditation and prayer, exercise, aerobics, martial arts. The important thing is to enjoy the activity for its own sake, and to know that what matters is not the result, but the control one is acquiring over one's attention." That's another Csikszentmihalyi special, and I was blown away when I read it because it's really at the core of how I feel about exercise. It's a way of focusing myself on the present moment and the activity at hand. Breathing. Putting one foot in front of the other. Picking the feet back up.

There Is No Such Thing as Drudgery.　"It is also important to develop the habit of doing whatever needs to be done with concentrated attention. Even the most routine tasks, like washing dishes, dressing, or mowing the lawn, become more rewarding if we approach them with the care it would take to make a work of art." I'm the usual dishwasher in our family because Tim is usually the cook, an arrangement that suits me very well. Sometimes I feel like getting those dishes clean is a drag, but other times I have a sense of craftsmanship and challenge: "How can I get these dishes as clean as possible with the minimum amount of wasted energy?" When you wash dishes old-fashioned way, this actually requires a certain amount of concentration and decision making. What gets rinsed in hot water before the sink is filled; what gets put to soak; what gets stacked on top of what in the sink. It is an art, if you let it be one.

FINDING FLOW THROUGH THE NOSE (NO, NOT LIKE THAT) WITH GUEST STAR LISA ENGLES

Because Lisa's brand of athletic guidance is as much about the brain as the body, I asked her for her number one tip for finding flow in movement. Her answer might surprise you:

"There's a powerful connection between the body and the mind. Over four thousand years ago, healers knew that breath affects our heart rate and our brain wave state. When you can control your breathing, you can automatically put yourself in an alpha state. That's what the runner's high is. Breathing can be used to alter your state of mind, and anybody can use it. One of the easiest ways to induce flow is to engage in nasal breathing. But it takes practice.

"The people I work with who are most receptive to nasal breathing are the people who are not conditioned to be 'athletes.' They find huge benefits. The elite athletes are the hardest to work with because you have to slow down at first to practice the breathing, and they don't want to slow down; it clashes with their egos. Nasal breathing requires strength in the diaphragm and the intercostal muscles in the ribs to expand and contract your chest wall and draw in the breath.

continues

Finding Flow Through the Nose *continued*

Nasal breathing stimulates the parasympathetic nervous system, putting your brain into a more relaxed state.

"Give yourself permission to have the experience of just breathing through your nose. Don't wear a watch or a heart rate monitor. Maybe try it once a week. Then maybe twice a week. It'll be a workout, but don't time yourself or make it your hardest session of the week." And yes, Lisa does mean to do this during a workout. It's good to breathe through your nose at other times too, but even during exercise, you can experiment with inhaling and exhaling with your mouth closed. Try doing it for a minute at a time at first, or even thirty seconds. It will seem like you're trying to suck wet concrete through a straw at first, but as you practice, your whole breathing apparatus (diaphragm, rib muscles, back, throat) will become more efficient at pulling in the air through the nose. If it seems too hard, just exercise less intensively.

If you hate it after about ten practice sessions, then quit. But really give it a try. Here's why: learning to breathe better equals learning to be a better athlete, period. You can train all you want, and that's great, but paying attention to your breathing is as important, if not more important, than anything else. You're not going anywhere without oxygen. The nose breathing practice is like a secret weapon in your arsenal. I've practiced it, and it does help you lower your heart rate and feel less stress during athletic endeavors.

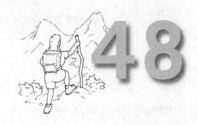

ENDURE

YOU MIGHT THINK that the injunction to endure would apply only to endurance sports. As a rule of thumb an endurance sport is one that lasts over an hour. Running, cycling, triathlon, long-distance swimming, cross-country skiing, and open water canoe racing come to mind right away. However, no matter what sport you choose to pursue in your imperfect way, it will require you to endure.

The English verb "to endure" comes from the Latin "indurare," which means "to harden" or "to make hard." The word took on the additional and related meaning "to last" and then, ominously, "to suffer." *Webster's* defines "endure" as "to remain firm under suffering or misfortune without yielding."

This is the connotation of endurance that puts people off exercise, especially the kind that goes on for a while. It hurts, people think, and the longer you do it, the more it hurts. Why else would all those late-night ads exist, the ones for exercise machines promising astonishing bodies in return for your practically painless investment of fifteen minutes a day?

But what if endurance wasn't painful? What if it was just a combination of how you perceive the sensations of your body in motion and how you set your mind to accept those sensations? Because the original meaning of "endure" just means to last. It doesn't contain any value judgments or imply suffering. It just means that you keep doing what you're doing.

But if you keep doing what you're doing for a long time and it involves movement, isn't that going to cause pain and suffering? Not necessarily. Say you aim to run a half marathon, 13.1 miles. As explained earlier in this book, you build up to it (and pretty much everything else) gradually, incrementally increasing the distances you can run each week, stepping back your mileage every few weeks to give yourself a chance to recover and consolidate your endurance gains. The key to your weekly long runs is to conduct them at a comfortable pace that you can maintain for a long time without breathing too hard, feeling burning in your legs, or experiencing other symptoms of suffering. If your breathing is ragged and your lungs are on fire, you are not doing that long run correctly. It's a far better approach to jog along easily for five or ten minutes, then take a little walk and stretch break for minute or so, then resume again at your easy pace. If you can't find an easy pace to be jogging at, you need to slow down. If you slow down to a walk, then that's just where you're at.

When you have built up a solid base of endurance over many weeks or months, then you might want to try shorter sessions of more intense effort, which can help build your speed. Notice here that I did not say, "Run as fast as you possibly can until you collapse." Depending on the kind of speed work you are doing, you may be running once around the track at a pace that makes your legs and lungs burn some, then resting until you are fully recovered, then doing that a few more times. The idea is to push your body a little bit for a short time, then let it recover, until it adapts to a different kind of workload. Is this suffering? I have referred to it that way, I admit. I remember standing bent over, hands on knees, sucking in huge gulps of air after a grueling 600-meter interval. Some people might think of that sensation as "pain," but that's just sissy talk.

It's not really pain. Not like pain when you stub your toe viciously on the leg of the coffee table or the oral surgeon hacks out your wisdom teeth. Those are traumas to the body that cause swelling and bleeding, whether internal or external. Running a little harder than you're used to is just a small stretch for your lungs and your heart, for your legs and your muscles, but most of all for your brain. It's not something your body's not meant to do, as much as you might mutter to yourself after each interval, "My body's not meant to do this." It is meant to do this. Exactly this.

Part of learning to endure, then, is recognizing what's real pain and what's just a "sensation of effort" as Coach Lisa likes to remind us in her infuriatingly chipper fashion. As you build up your foundation of exercise experience and your body learns to adapt to the new requests you're making of it, those sensations of effort will not be as unpleasant as you thought the first time you experienced them. And that brings me, with grand rhetorical flourish, to another definition of "endure": "to regard with acceptance or tolerance." So regard your exercise with acceptance and tolerance. Accept that various levels of effort make your body feel certain ways. Study your responses. Learn how to push yourself without crossing that line into real pain. Accept your effort.

Learn to endure and learn to love it.

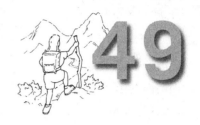

KNOW WHEN TO QUIT

SOMETIMES QUITTING IS your best option. Oh golly, I know that sounds un-American of me, not to mention wimpy. We heap adulation on nonquitters in sports and life, on those who struggle through to the finish, no matter what the cost. In 1982 Julie Moss brought worldwide attention to the Ironman triathlon by wobbling, stumbling, falling, and finally crawling the final few yards across the finish line. A true hero, the commentators said, the very ideal of persistence and determination. From an emotional and psychological perspective, it's hard to disagree. Seeing that footage of Julie willing herself across the finish line still gives me goosebumps.

After seeing that footage, though, would you wonder about the cost weeks or months down the line? Is draining your body's energy to the point where your legs stop responding to your brain's commands really the best investment of your hard-won fitness resources? Well, for Julie Moss, leading the Ironman with one hundred yards to go, it seemed like a good idea. Earlier in the race, though, because she tried to keep running rather than walking, she ended up not being able to do either and was reduced to crawling. She was passed by Kathleen Mc-Cartney seconds before reaching the line. Almost nobody now remembers Kathleen McCartney, the 1982 Ironman women's champion. Julie Moss, on the other hand, is a legend who didn't quit. But as Vince Lombardi would point out, she didn't win, either.

I would not have advised Julie to quit at those last hundred yards. By the time you start falling down, you've already gone way into the red zone, beyond what your body can tolerate, and you've stayed there so long that those extra yards wouldn't make much difference. But I think that when you are in an event or even a training session where you are in far over your head, badly prepared, or sick, and it just feels wrong to continue, there should be no shame in abandoning the field.

Let's not get delusions of grandeur here. Most who are reading this book are in no danger of being passed in the final ten yards of Ironman Hawaii and losing the overall women's title by seconds. Finishing an Ironman, maybe. Finishing an Ironman with a whole hour to spare before the mandatory seventeen-hour time cutoff, even better. Finishing a half Ironman—just fine too.

For imperfect athletes, strategic quitting is often something to consider. Even if it's a training session where you just feel like crap. You've waited till you know you're good and warmed up because sometimes it's just that first half-hour where you feel awful; once you get your blood flowing and your muscles warmed up, things are okay. Well, that didn't work, so you've eased off your intensity, opting to go along slowly until you feel better. However, you still feel horrid. Not just tired, but tired in your bones. You've checked your hydration and nutrition, and you're not low on fluids or blood sugar, but your legs (or whatever bits of you are working hardest) just feel dead. Maybe you feel nause-ated, or your body aches all over. Or maybe you have this pain in your knee that seems to be getting worse. This would be a good time for a strategic quit. Maybe you haven't been getting enough sleep or leaving enough recovery time between challenging ex-ercise sessions. You may have been ramping up your activity too quickly. STOP. Just stop. Go home and take a nap. Live to fight another day.

You may not get to win the Ironman this way, but you have a better chance of making it to the start line of your big event without getting injured or sick. Don't let your ego push you into something that's going to hurt you down the line. Some-times this can be hard, especially when you're training with other people. Even if they're not busting on you for quitting, you bust on yourself for even considering it. Ignore that feeling.

But what if you are actually at your big event and you start feeling this way? What if all your training, all your preparation, all your hours of work and play lead you to the starting line and you feel like crap? Or what if you get a nasty case of the runs halfway through the race or sprain your knee in the second round of the tae kwon do tournament? Do you forge on or do you quit?

I can't tell you what to do here. You have to evaluate the whole situation. How important is the event to you? What does your body feel? Does it really feel smart to go on? Is there an-other event in two months that you can aim for instead? Are you risking months of recovery or rehab for a few hours that you have designated in your mind as extremely special? Or are you going to put everything on the line, no matter what the cost? It's your call. Consider it carefully, as dispassionately as you can, and in consultation with people who know more than you do. This won't always be possible, but when you can, check with medics along the course. Big events that are hard will have them. If you have a coach you can check in with, do it. Often a friend or family member among the spectators can offer you a slightly more objective opinion on how messed up you are.

Maybe you'll get over the runs and finish the race without further incident. Maybe you'll get dehydrated and end up in the first aid tent with an IV needle in your arm, or even in the hospital overnight. Maybe your knee is just twisted and will hold up for two more rounds of competition, or maybe you've put a slight tear in the ligament that the next round will exacerbate, ending your athletic career for six months to a year.

Sometimes, quitting is the way to go. And just to keep the ghost of Coach Lombardi off my back, I have to say that I am not advocating quitting on your big picture dreams. Those are not quittable. And don't quit just because you feel kind of tired, or you're scared you can't do it, or you feel like you won't do well. Quitting should only happen when not quitting endangers your health and/or your big picture dreams. It's another tool in your arsenal. Use it wisely.

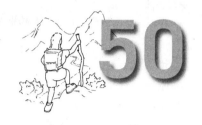

DEVELOP THE
FULL-BODY SCAN

I WANT TO talk about how you can get seriously into the flow by tuning into your body. This may involve backing away from your iPod, which I know is a controversial piece of advice. I know many, many aspiring athletes for whom exercise without the iPod (or other MP3 player, if you insist) would seem like a form of torture. The iPod is so perfect: so convenient, so tiny, so full of peppy and inspiring music, so beautifully designed. What could possibly be wrong with taking the iPod along on your athletic adventures?

Well, nothing's wrong with it, as such. I own an iPod. Recently, as I've been trying to get my running going again after months of illness and nagging injuries, I've put the iPod on to distract myself from how slow I am and how lacking in stamina compared to last year.

But that's the thing. The iPod distracts me. And I suspect it distracts you too. "But," you say, "I want to be distracted. That's the whole point!" You may look at Chapter 47 and say that the music helps you find flow. And you might be right. I would contend, however, that you're getting into a music-induced flow, rather than an exercise-induced flow. I have a hypothesis that if you're in music-based flow, chugging along, with all your focus on the tunes, I figure you're not giving your movement and your athletic development the concentrated attention that our bud Mihalyi writes about. You're not seeking that optimal balance of challenge and skills, where you're stretching your perceived limits just enough to keep you fully engaged. You're fully engaged with the B-52s or Verdi or My Chemical Romance or Johnny Cash. You may be improving yourself as an appreciator of music, but I don't think you're improving yourself as an athlete. Or your improvement, if any, is less than it would be if your attention were on how you're moving.

It's totally fine if your focus isn't on improving as an athlete. If you're contented with your current level of imperfection and just want to use your exercise time to do double duty with your music appreciation time, that's cool. What matters most is that you're moving and that you're enjoying it. Period.

Suppose, though, that one of the reasons you bought this book is that you want to, well, kick some butt. It doesn't have to be someone else's butt; the butt you kick can just as easily be your own. "Kicking butt" is just another way to say "getting better." So if you want to get better at your sport of choice, it might behoove you to pay close attention to what you're doing. It's hard to get better at anything without paying close attention to it.

Paying close attention can be fun and rewarding. Yoga encourages it "through the medium of the breath," as they like to say. You pay attention to your muscles and joints by mentally sending your breath to them. Some advanced physical training regimens have you think about a muscle, touch a muscle, think about moving it, and then actually move it.

Or you can do something as simple yet rewarding as a full-body scan without stopping what you're doing. This useful process, which you perform during your exercise, involves devoting a few seconds of attention to each part of your body, starting with your toes, moving to the balls of your feet, to your arches, your heels, your ankles, shins, knees, and so on. Move up your legs to your hips and butt, your abdomen, low back, all the way up to the top of your head.

Name your body parts to yourself, toes, arches, knees, shoulders. As you undertake a more detailed study of your functional anatomy, you might find yourself scanning your Achilles tendon, your quadriceps, your trapezius muscles, and your transversus abdominus.

Notice how each body part is feeling. Is there tension? Is there chafing? Is there fatigue or sharp pain? And be open to positive sensations too. Is there strength? Is there fluidity? Is there relaxation?

Once you've run through the parts, start again from the bottom or work back down from the top, and send a positive thought to each part. "My knees are strong; the joints work smoothly. My thighs are powerful." Whatever works for you. It's amazing how this little exercise can pass the time and infuse you with new energy.

Once you're done with that, you can concentrate on your breathing for a while. Keep it in a steady rhythm, in sync with your movement. Then you can count foot speed, number of right foot strikes per minute, or cadence if you're cycling. You can focus on snapping off your right jabs if you're working with the heavy bag. Then check in with yourself to see if you need some fluid or food, especially if you've been having fun in this way for a while.

After a while, you get to the point where you're so busy noticing your body and its miraculous workings that you're not really noticing either the music you have in your earbuds or the discomfort or boredom you were trying to banish with the music. This process can be, if you will allow me the indulgence, a very powerful spiritual experience, a union with the present moment and the infinity of possibility that the moment represents. Just you, your breath, your body, and the universe. Check it out.

AFTERWORD
Find Your Own Path

OKAY, **READERS,** that is pretty much all I know and most of what I believe about making yourself the happiest athlete you can be. The last thing I want to tell you is this: find your own way. I have my own experience. I have what I've read, and the things I've talked about with other athletes, both accomplished and struggling. But you are the authority on what works for you.

If self-consciousness works for you and makes you a better person and a happier athlete, hey, rock on. If you think it's positively disgusting to sweat anywhere or at any time, whether there's a person within fifty miles of you or not, that's absolutely your prerogative. If the whole reason you exercise is so you can listen to your iPod, awesome. Maybe you think it's dorky to imagine yourself as a superhero. Hmm, probably so. There is no one way to work this.

Come up with your own list of tips and tricks that make you a better athlete. They might include some of the things in this book. My old friend Russ always savors some beer when he gets home from a hard race, whereas drinking beer after running makes my legs hurt. Russ's list would almost certainly include "Have a Beer. Or Two"; mine would not. Not that I have anything against beer. Far from it. Your list might include "Make Sure Your Feet Are Pretty," and that would be very valid. Actually, maybe I should add that one, though it's a bit late now. Pretty feet, free of calluses and dead skin, are less prone to blistering, and they make you feel fast.

You are the ultimate arbiter of your own approach to your sport or sports. It has to work for you. You need to think about yourself, the things that make you happy, the things that you think make you unhappy and whether that's real unhappiness or just fear of the unknown. You need to think about what makes you feel competitive, if anything, and whether that competitiveness is fun for you or makes you feel all knotted up and anxious. And then you need to devise your set of principles and practices to guide you along your journey, whether you follow them all the time or just most of the time. You may make some mistakes along the way. One of my sports heroes, John Wooden, who led his UCLA basketball teams to an unequaled ten national championships, didn't win his first national title until his sixteenth year at UCLA. That's a lot of mistakes. But Coach Wooden eventually learned to embrace his mistakes: "If you're not making mistakes, then you're not doing anything."

Books are useful, certainly, as are websites, coaches, peers, teams, clubs, and clinics. But if you end up following one training program or another with slavish devotion, then I'll be sad because any book or website or even coach that claims to have the one true way to athletic nirvana is full of crap. You have to be the one who decides what feels right for your body, your mind, and your spirit. It's your game. You make the rules, and ultimately you decide what success is.

If you've been on a journey to shaping up for a while now, I hope that you've found a few morsels of thought to chew on, digest, and use to fuel yourself as you keep on going. If you're new to the idea of moving yourself around for the purpose of enjoyment and fitness, you've got a great ride in front of you. Pick one small thing I talk about in these pages, and do me a favor. Go out and do it tomorrow.

ACKNOWLEDGMENTS

Shape Up with the Slow Fat Triathlete would not have existed without the contributions and inspiration of my fellow "imperfect athletes:" Rebecca Bailey, Indigo Brude, Leslie Clavey, Bonnie Crawford, Dana Kelly, Russ Kiel, Nadya Lawson, Kelly McIntyre, Michelle Oakes, Anne Nesbet, Pat Silver, Paula Stout, Mary Jane Zanelli. These few, these happy few, this band of sisters—they rock. They represent the millions of imperfect athletes and soon-to-be imperfect athletes who are the reason I wrote this book. They run, they sail, they hike, they kickbox, they dance, they do yoga, they play volleyball, they complete Ironman triathlons, they endure. They have way too much fun.

Huge piles of gratitude to the more expert athletes, coaches, and writers who weighed in with their experience, advice, and encouragement for me and all my readers: Bad Bob Baker, who makes ultra-distance cross-country skiing sound like a jolly time; Jeanette De Patie, the aerobics instructor we all wish we could have had for our first aerobics class; the incomparable Sally Edwards, triathlon and fitness hero and the prophet of heart rate-based training; Petra Eggert, who has treated my bones and muscles and kept me moving forward; Lisa Engles, who puts the "personal" in personal trainer and the fun into exercise; Beth Rypins, whitewater champion and the queen of questioning assumptions; Dan Sauers, mental toughness consultant and coach of tri newbies; Suzanne Schlosberg, who has figured out more and funnier ways to say "eat less, exercise more" than any woman on the planet; Rocky Snyder, who can be my guru any day; and Kyle Welch, who demonstrates daily that fabulous athleticism and fabulous kindness can and do go hand in hand.

The aforementioned Anne Nesbet is my patron saint of perseverance and confidant about all things writing. David Dahl is my home-grown yet powerful agent. Renée Sedliar is the editor who is responsible for any coherence this book may demonstrate. Extra helpings of gratitude to this table.

Any errors that I have made in conveying the knowledge, wisdom, humor, and insight of everyone who has helped me become the Slow Fat Triathlete are entirely my own.

INDEX

259